A REPORT ON RESEARCHES
ON SPRUE IN CEYLON
1912—1914

A REPORT ON RESEARCHES
ON SPRUE IN CEYLON
1912—1914

BY

P. H. BAHR

M.A., M.D., D.T.M. and H. (Cantab.), M.R.C.P. (Lond.), M.R.C.S.

London School of Tropical Medicine
Horton-Smith prizeman, Cambridge, 1914

Cambridge :
at the University Press
1915

CAMBRIDGE
UNIVERSITY PRESS

University Printing House, Cambridge CB2 8BS, United Kingdom

Cambridge University Press is part of the University of Cambridge.

It furthers the University's mission by disseminating knowledge in the pursuit of education, learning and research at the highest international levels of excellence.

www.cambridge.org
Information on this title: www.cambridge.org/9781107492943

© Cambridge University Press 1915

First published 1915
Re-issued 2015

A catalogue record for this publication is available from the British Library

ISBN 978-1-107-49294-3 Paperback

Cambridge University Press has no responsibility for the persistence or accuracy of URLs for external or third-party internet websites referred to in this publication, and does not guarantee that any content on such websites is, or will remain, accurate or appropriate.

....

Every effort has been made in preparing this book to provide accurate and up-to-date information which is in accord with accepted standards and practice at the time of publication. Although case histories are drawn from actual cases, every effort has been made to disguise the identities of the individuals involved. Nevertheless, the authors, editors and publishers can make no warranties that the information contained herein is totally free from error, not least because clinical standards are constantly changing through research and regulation. The authors, editors and publishers therefore disclaim all liability for direct or consequential damages resulting from the use of material contained in this book. Readers are strongly advised to pay careful attention to information provided by the manufacturer of any drugs or equipment that they plan to use.

PREFACE

IN the following pages I have recounted a rather laborious attempt to unravel the etiology of one of the least understood, but nevertheless one of the most insidious diseases known to Tropical Medicine.

Although the final results of this investigation cannot be regarded as conclusive, yet it is hoped that they are of some value and may serve as a basis for future investigators in other localities where sprue is indigenous.

P. H. BAHR.

PRESCOT, LANCS.
March 1915.

CONTENTS

APPENDICES

LIST OF ILLUSTRATIONS

CHAPTER I

ORIGIN AND OBJECTS OF THE EXPEDITION

THE frequent occurrence during recent years of sprue amongst the planting community of Ceylon, together with the lack of trust-worthy information on the subject, made it advisable, from an economic, as well as from a humanitarian point of view, that the subject should be investigated in the light of modern research.

Sir Patrick Manson had for some time past been in correspondence[1] on the subject with Sir Henry Macallum, G.C.M.G., the late Governor of the Colony, with the result that the Legislative Council voted £750 towards such an investigation and a further sum of £250 was provided for the same object by the executors of the late Mr E. S. Grigson, a former chairman of the Planters' Association, and himself a victim of the disease.

Accordingly the Committee of the London School of Tropical Medicine was requested to elect a representative to undertake this work and the author of the present paper was selected for the purpose.

I arrived in the Colony on March 16th 1912 and left on June 3rd 1913, having collected a considerable amount of information and pathological material bearing on sprue which I have since worked out, by kind permission of the authorities, at the London School of Tropical Medicine. For the seven months subsequent to my return from Ceylon I was continuously engaged in this work, in which I have been assisted throughout by my excellent assistant Mr W. J. Muggleton, who had accompanied me on a similar mission in 1910–11 to Fiji. In Ceylon a laboratory was installed on the back verandah of a private bungalow which I leased in Nuwara Eliya, a town situated at an elevation of 6200 ft. My reasons for selecting this town as the headquarters of the research were founded on the fact that it is the chief sanatorium of the Colony, to which invalids tend to gravitate, and whence all plantations and districts of the island can easily be reached by downhill road. Nuwara Eliya has the further advantage that the temperature is such (the thermometer rarely registering more than 75° F.) as to admit of prolonged physical and mental exertions.

---

[1] For correspondence on this subject, see *Year Book of the Planters' Association of Ceylon*, 1912, pp. 2, 8, 20, 35–36, 41, 100, 166–173.

CHAPTER II

ACKNOWLEDGMENTS

I NEED hardly say that the efforts of a private individual in a research of this kind, in Ceylon, would be of little avail, were he not actively supported by the Government authorities, and the Planters' Association, both of which took a great interest in the work, and assisted me in every way in their power.

I am therefore much indebted to Sir Allan Perry, the principal civil medical officer, and to Dr G. Rutherford, who acted while the former was on leave, for having given me every facility in the hospitals under their charge.

It would be invidious to single out any individual District Medical Officer to whom my thanks are due; without exception they unreservedly permitted me to examine their cases and to perform postmortems in the district hospitals. I, however, especially wish to express my thanks to Dr F. Grenier, Physician to the Colombo General Hospital. I have also been greatly assisted by many private practitioners, especially Dr R. J. Drummond, late of Talawakelle, Ceylon, who has had a considerable experience of sprue in its early stages.

Mr E. Burgess, assistant at the Bacteriological Institute, Colombo, has assisted me in ways too numerous to mention.

Finally, I must acknowledge the unfailing advice and encouragement afforded me throughout this enquiry by Sir Patrick Manson, G.C.M.G., F.R.S., especially during the four months December 1912 to March 1913 when he visited the Colony, and also by Dr C. W. Daniels, of the London School of Tropical Medicine.

Every effort was made to visit all the planting districts of the island, especially those in which several cases of the disease had occurred and to interview past and present victims of the disease. Any success I may have attained in this way is entirely due to the unreserved manner in which many private individuals entrusted me with the history of their illnesses.

Such necessary laboratory apparatus as an incubator, autoclave, etc. with which I was unprovided were loaned to me by the Medical Department, while I was also permitted to buy drugs and reagents at cost price.

CHAPTER III

A DESCRIPTION OF CEYLON, ITS INHABITANTS, VEGETATION, GEOLOGY AND PREVALENT DISEASES

ALTHOUGH it is difficult to compress into a reasonable space a description of Ceylon, I think it is essential in a report of this nature that I should describe briefly the physical features of the country inasmuch as they seem to bear upon the epidemiology of sprue. The island is situated between latitude 5·59′ and 9·51′ N. and longitude 79·41′ and 81·54′ E. and is separated from India by a channel 40 miles wide, a distance almost spanned by the island of Mannar and the series of coral reefs forming Adam's Bridge. It measures about 270 miles from north to south and about 140 miles in its greatest width, and occupies an area of about 25,481 square miles (equal to that of Holland and Belgium) and supports a population slightly over 4,000,000 (about equal to that of Ireland).

As to four-fifths, the island is an undulating plain, the coastal zone surrounds a central mountainous area of considerable elevation and of singular beauty. The central mountainous plateau, about 4000 square miles, is situated towards the south and is almost equidistant from the east and west coasts. Across this central mountainous region from north to south runs a dividing range. This range is composed of some 150 mountains of from 3700 ft. to 8296 ft. in height; Pidurutugalla and Adam's Peak are the best known and most prominent of these.

None of the rivers in Ceylon are navigable by ships, and only a few by boats. The largest river, the Mahaweliganga, rises in the heart of the mountains and flows into the sea at Trincomalee on the east coast after a course of 200 miles.

The mountainous country is provided with many beautiful rushing torrents, which in many instances have been successfully stocked with trout, indicating a comparatively low temperature.

The population represents a considerable number of races. This results from the fact that several European as well as Asiatic nations have in turn occupied the country. The Portuguese settled on the west and south coasts in 1507 and were dispossessed by the Dutch 150 years later. They in turn yielded to the English in 1796. As

1—2

a result of the several invasions by Asiatic tribes some seventy-eight races are to-day represented in the island. We need concern ourselves here only with the most prominent types.

The Sinhalese, a people peculiar to Ceylon, of Aryan race and originating from the north of India, form the bulk of the population and number over 2,700,000. They are divided into two classes, the low-country and the up-country or Kandyan. The former are twice as numerous as the latter. Although a considerable number are Christians the large majority are Buddhists. Their language is akin to Sanskrit.

The Veddas, a people also peculiar to Ceylon, and supposed to represent a pre-Aryan indigenous population, are but a small element in the population, numbering only about 5000. The remnant of this race still wanders in the jungles of the Eastern Province tracking and hunting their game with primitive bow and arrow.

The Tamils, who number over 1,000,000, are of Dravidian stock. They came to Ceylon in two ways: centuries ago as invaders and conquerors, and are still coming in at the rate of 100,000 annually imported as labourers from S. India. The descendants of the early Tamils, a fine manly race, are known as Ceylon Tamils, and live principally in the Northern and Eastern Provinces, where their language mostly prevails.

The Moors, who number some 260,000, are of Arab origin. On account of their religion—Mohammedanism—they live somewhat aloof from the other races. They are generally traders and for the most part speak the Tamil language.

The Burghers, about 26,000 in number, are of Portuguese, Dutch, and English descent. The higher classes fill the learned professions and many are engaged in mercantile pursuits or are members of the Civil Service.

The Malays, who are Mohammedans, are chiefly descended from soldiers imported from the Malay Peninsula. They fill the ranks of the police and find positions as prison warders, office messengers, etc.

Besides these races, there are numbers of tall savage-looking Afghans, familiar and picturesque figures in their flowing robes. They are usually usurers and horse dealers. Kaffirs of mixed blood, descended from soldiers imported by the Dutch in olden times, are occasionally met with.

For administrative purposes, Ceylon is divided into nine Provinces. Of these the Western is by far the most thickly populated, having 721 persons to the square mile. Next to it in density of population and in prosperity is the great tea-bearing mountainous area of the Central Province, with 172 persons to the square mile. The North-Eastern Province, by far the largest in extent, is the least densely populated; it has but 21 persons to the square mile. This arid deserted country, now known as the "Wanni," was once, many hundred years before the Christian era, populated by thousands of the wonderful race who have left behind them as monuments to their skill and civilisation the ruined cities of Anuradhapura and Polonnurua besides hundreds of gigantic irrigation tanks.

The Europeans, who number about 7500, not including the military, naval and merchant marine services, are mostly confined to the plantations of the Central Province and to the Colombo district. There are but few Europeans in the Northern, North-Central, and Eastern Provinces.

The climate. It has been said that considering its size no country has such a variety of climate as Ceylon. The only feature common to all parts is the slight variation in the climatic elements in any given place.

Health in Ceylon depends in great measure on the elevation, rainfall, and cultivation. In the hilly districts, at an altitude of 1500 feet or over, the climate is healthy considering it is a tropical one. In the low-country, it is hot and unhealthy.

The mean annual rainfall varies from 30 to 40 inches in the north to 200 inches in the interior of the island. There are two seasons in Ceylon, the south-west and north-east monsoons. During the former, rainfall is confined mostly to the south-west part of the island, during the latter the rains are more evenly distributed throughout the entire island.

The south-west monsoon is said to commence at the beginning of April, reaching its height in the middle of May, and ending about the middle of August, when the north-east monsoon sets in accompanied by heavy rains which last till January.

The island may be divided into two dry and three wet zones. The dry zones—north and east—embracing about two-thirds of the island, receive less than 75 inches of rain per annum. As most of this rain falls within two months it is comparatively useless for agriculture, unless when artificially stored in tanks. The more fertile portions of the island are contained within the three wet zones—central, west and south. The first of these (rainfall 75–200 inches) comprises all the best tea and cocoa estates.

The temperature varies with the elevation and the seasons from an average mean of less than 60° F. in Nuwara Eliya to over 80° F. in the hot low-country districts and in Colombo.

Vegetation. The flora is as varied as the climate and comprises over three thousand species of flowering plants and ferns. The low-country is one of the most highly cultivated districts, the valley bottoms being occupied chiefly by rice fields. The more elevated ground being covered with the characteristic mixed cultivation of the Sinhalese, such as the jackfruit, the breadfruit, coconut, areca, mango, plantain, yam, custard apple, toddy palm, betel, pepper and other small plants. Large areas along the sea coast and along the Kandy railway are given up to coconut cultivation.

The low-country cultivation conducted by Europeans is mainly found in the Kelani Valley and the Kalutara districts. The principal products are tea of a poor quality, but of a large yield, and in the lower districts, rubber, which is gradually ousting tea from its premier position. Cocoa, cloves, nutmeg, vanilla and other crops are also grown as high up to Kandy (1700 ft.). Higher up among the hills the climate becomes colder and less sunny, and the more tropical forms of vegetation, as palms and the larger bamboos, gradually disappear. So much land has been taken up for tea cultivation that very little is now left of the vast forests of evergreen shrubs which clothed the mountain zone. Fearing a serious diminution in the rainfall, as a consequence of these extensive clearings, the Government no longer sells land above 5000 ft. so as to conserve the primitive jungle above that line and thus to assure an adequate rainfall.

Rice and other native cultivations cease above about 2000 ft. From this to 5000 ft. tea is the prominent feature, as was coffee in days gone by.

The lack of native timber is supplied by the planting on the tea estates of vast numbers of Australian trees, especially the silky oak (*Albizzia*), the *Grevillea* and many species of *Eucalyptus*.

At the highest levels and on the Horton Plains, and to eastward over the main watershed, the jungle is broken by patches of grass lands, known as " Patanas," covered with a turf of rank grass.

To the north-west, north, east, and south-west of the mountains there lies a vast plain, the dry zone. The climate of this zone is like that of Southern India, and the vegetation is similar. With the re-establishment of the ancient systems of irrigation in this area tobacco planting is becoming a large industry.

Geology. The geological strata of the greater part of Ceylon consist of gneiss and metamorphic rocks, especially characterised by variability in their composition. They are to be regarded for the most part as of igneous origin, though it is possible that some metamorphic sedimentary rocks also exist; the former are known as granulites or gneisses, and belong to the Charnockite series of South India. The red soil of the tea and rubber plantations is formed mostly of weathered ferruginous and micaceous gneiss.

Prevalent diseases. Amongst the European population probably typhoid, amoebic dysentery, malaria and sprue are the most common diseases. The two former account for the most deaths, typhoid being specially prevalent in Colombo. Bacillary dysentery occurs sporadically, chiefly in young children (the Y bacillus of Hiss and Russell was the one most commonly isolated by me).

Amongst the native population malaria and ankylostomiasis are very prevalent. The latter claims a great number of victims especially among the plantation labourers, being found in an aggravated form in many low-lying estates, though its effects are often evident in the up-country coolies as well. Malaria, I have good reason to believe, rarely originates *de novo* above 2500 feet, but is a veritable scourge in the low-lying districts and of the rubber and coconut plantations in the Southern Province.

Diarrhoea figures largely in official reports as a cause of death among coolies. It is probably a symptom of a variety of different diseases, of which the ankylostome and the dysentery amoeba are among the commonest of the exciting causes.

Yaws is very prevalent among the Sinhalese in the dry Northern and Eastern districts, but is not found at all in the higher altitudes. Syphilis is very common among the Tamil labourers and is a great scourge. The death rate of the Colony is a high one and seems to be on the increase. In 1905 it was 35·1 per thousand; in 1912 it is said to have stood at a higher figure. The birth rate has increased of late years and in 1911 was at 39 per thousand.

CHAPTER IV

A DEFINITION OF SPRUE AND A DESCRIPTION OF
ITS SYMPTOMS

SPRUE is a disease, essentially of the tropics. It is characterised by symptoms suggestive of a chronic affection of the alimentary tract and of the glandular organs subserving digestion.

The disease rarely runs an acute course, usually its progress is subject to periods of quiescence and exacerbation; it may remain latent even for a number of years.

In typical cases the tongue presents at first a peculiar raw appearance, most marked at the tip and edges, due to inflammation of the fungiform papillae. This process eventually leads to atrophy of all the papillae and to an eroded condition of the entire mucous surface of the mouth. Associated with these changes small yellow aphthous ulcers often appear periodically on the tongue and the buccal mucosa, especially on the inner surface of the lower lip, the cheeks, the fraenum or the soft palate.

Flatulent dyspepsia is generally a marked feature and is accompanied by distension of the entire intestinal canal, particularly of the small intestine. This distension is only relieved by the frequent passage, especially in the early morning, of large, pale, frothy acid stools and of much flatus.

In many instances the inflammatory disturbance spreads down the oesophagus, causing great pain and difficulty of swallowing; there may be, and usually is, extreme hyperaesthesia of the mouth parts, and the sense of taste is often in abeyance. In the later and profoundly anaemic stage there is a tendency to patchy pigmentation between the scapulae and on the interior aspect of the thighs.

Symptoms persisting, atrophy of all the organs of the body, particularly of the liver, and profound anaemia ensue. The disease unless promptly and properly treated ultimately proves fatal.

CHAPTER V

HILL DIARRHOEA

As in the sequel frequent reference will be made to hill diarrhoea, a disease which in some respects resembles sprue and which is frequently associated and confused with sprue, a word on the subject seems desirable.

Grant in 1854 first described the hill diarrhoea occurring at Simla at an elevation of 6500–8000 feet. He indicated it as a cause of serious inefficiency and loss to the English troops stationed there, and regarded the disease as a manifestation of scurvy. Crombie in 1880 described a very severe epidemic in Simla in which about 75 per cent. of the population were attacked. He regarded the disease as a functional disorder of the liver, brought about by the unaccustomed low temperature of the high altitudes, due to previous residence in the hot plains of India. Duncan advanced the hypothesis that this peculiar form of diarrhoea was due to the presence of mica in the drinking water derived from the laterite rocks. His hypothesis was revived and supported by Dyson, though Crombie in the Simla epidemic had excluded water as a factor.

Hill diarrhoea appears not to be limited to the hill stations of India; a similar affection is said to occur in the highlands of Europe, S. Africa and S. America. It is apt to occur in epidemics which observe a distinct seasonal character in their occurrence. Like sprue it is characterised by flatulent dyspepsia accompanied by nausea and sometimes vomiting, by the passage of large, liquid, pale and fermenting stools and by the marked tendency of this diarrhoea to occur in the early morning. In the early stages of the illness the stools are said to be dark coloured and bilious.

Its differentiation from sprue rests principally on clinical grounds. Amongst these may be mentioned the acuteness of the onset of hill diarrhoea, the absence of tongue symptoms, of toxaemia or of any appreciable shrinkage of the liver. In the majority of cases symptoms promptly subside on the patient leaving the endemic area for the plains; it is attended by little or no mortality. Sometimes diarrhoea persists for a considerable time and in a few instances may develop into, or predispose to, genuine sprue.

Though all classes and races are liable to attack, adult Europeans, especially visitors from the hot and low-lying districts, are most prone to contract the disorder. Children appear to be rarely attacked.

The facts, so far as they are known, rather suggest that hill diarrhoea is usually a functional disturbance of the digestive organs. Against this supposition, the experience of recent years has shown that there has been a decrease in the incidence of hill diarrhoea, apparently supervening on improvements in the sanitation and water supply of the Indian hill stations, a fact suggestive of some specific infection.

CHAPTER VI

THE TERM "SPRUE"

THE term "Sprue" has long been in use in the Netherland Indies as indicating forms of chronic diarrhoea, in the main that form which is the subject of this Report. It was first introduced into English medical literature by Manson in 1870 who anglicised the word into "Sprue[1]." About the same time the name was independently adopted in its Dutch form "Spruw" by Van der Burg. Previously to this, Bosch, in 1837, had applied it rather indefinitely to a variety of diarrhoeas.

To prevent confusion, it may be well to mention that this grave tropical disease has nothing to do with the aphthous stomatitis of badly-fed cachetic children, which was at one time known in Scotland and Holland as "Sprue" or "Spruw." They appear to be totally different conditions.

---

[1] Many names have been bestowed on the disease now known throughout the world as sprue. The following is approximately a correct list:

Aphthoides chronica—impetigo primarum viarum (Hillary, 1766); Indische spruw, aphthae tropicae (Van der Burg, 1880); sprue (Manson, 1880); psilosis linguae vel mucosae intestini (Thin, 1897). Up to about the last quarter of the 19th century it was known to Indian physicians as white flux, white purging, white chronic diarrhoea, diarrhoea alba, scorbutic diarrhoea, endemic entero-colitis, chronic enteritis of Indo-China, endemic diarrhoea of warm countries.

Amongst its rarer designations are the following: Ceylon sore mouth, Singapore sore mouth, cachexia aphthosa, stomatitis intertropica, aphthae orientalis, aphthaeo-gastro-enteritis tropicae, gastro-enteritis aphthae indica—phlegmasia membranae mucosae gastro-pulmonalis. In German it is generally called aphthae tropicae, in French athrepsie coloniale atrophique, in Dutch Indische spruw, in Malay seriawan (Carnegie-Brown), and in Sinhalese mandan or grahaney (Wijesakere).

CHAPTER VII

SUMMARY OF THE PAST LITERATURE OF SPRUE

THE earliest description of a disease in every respect corresponding with sprue was undoubtedly the one given by Hillary in his *Observations on the changes of air and concomitant epidemical diseases in the Island of Barbados*, in 1766.

Objections may be made to the applicability to sprue of his description on the ground of the rarity (judging from the modern records) of the disease in the West Indies and of the undoubted prevalence at the present day in several of these islands, notably Barbados where Hillary worked, of a pellagrous disease, the "psilosis pigmentosa[1]" of Cuthbert Bowen; an affection in which wasting, intense anaemia, pigmented patches on the hands and feet combined with a denuded tongue and uncontrollable diarrhoea, are the most prominent symptoms. Hillary, however, makes no mention of the pigmentation and mental symptoms— so frequent a feature in pellagra.

The writings of the Indian army surgeons of the last century contain many references to the diarrhoeas so prevalent in that country. A proportion of the cases they quote were in all probability of the nature of true sprue. Too much stress must not be laid on the clinical symptoms alone, however accurate; diagnosis in the absence of demonstration of the germ cause of these diseases is unreliable. Even at the present day, although the aetiological *rôles* of the dysentery amoeba and of the dysentery bacillus are more or less understood, we know little or nothing of the germ causes of the diarrhoeas, including that of sprue, of warm countries.

In 1829 Twining makes reference to a diarrhoea occurring amongst Europeans of long residence clinically characterised by pale copious stools, and pathologically by attenuation of the small intestine, but he makes no reference to the condition of the mouth.

Grant in 1854 described an already referred to diarrhoea which from its limitation to certain hill stations in India he termed "hill diarrhoea" or "diarrhoea alba." From his descriptions one is led to believe that a proportion of his cases was genuine sprue.

---

[1] C. J. Manning (1907): *Report on certain cases of Psilosis pigmentosa in Lunatic Asylums of Barbados.*

It is open to doubt whether up to 1881, when Sir Joseph Fayrer published his *Lettsomian Lectures* and made definite allusion to the mouth symptoms, sprue had been recognised in India as a clinical entity.

The French, after their occupation of Annam, had extensive opportunities of studying the diarrhoeas all too prevalent amongst their troops there, but it has been admitted that the writings of Julien, Dutrulau, Layet, Le Roy de Méricourt and others convey the idea, that sprue was merely a form of chronic dysentery. The writings of Bonnet, Mahé, Berenger-Feraud, on the other hand, seem to indicate that these authors, basing their statements on histo-pathological studies, regarded the diarrhoea of Cochin-China rather as a complication of, or as a sequel to, dysentery.

Then follows the elaborate studies of Kelsch and Kiener, and more especially the careful description of " entero-colite endemique des pays chauds" of Bertrand and Fontan, who, though writing with a full knowledge of Manson and Van der Burg's work, did not shed much further light on the subject, save to strengthen the idea that a considerable proportion of these Cochin-China cases tallies with the disease we now know as sprue. In 1888 Roux came to the same conclusion as Manson and Van der Burg and regarded sprue as distinct from dysentery.

The old Dutch authorities, though their works are little known, had written extensively of the diseases observed in their East Indian possessions; thus in 1837 we find Bosch referring under the name of " Indische spruw " to a chronic diarrhoea occurring amongst Europeans in Java and which he wished to ascribe to the effects of the climate and unsuitable diet. Waitz and Dozy in 1854 appeared to confuse the disease with dysentery, but in 1859 and again in 1873 Greiner referred to a diarrhoea of Java, in which he believed hereditary disposition played a part, under the name of " aphthae tropicae " which can be none other than the disease later so well described by his compatriot, Van der Burg.

The first definite accounts of sprue as a distinct and separate disease were written quite independently by Van der Burg in Java and by Manson in Amoy, China.

In his short paper published in the Medical Reports of the Chinese Customs Services, Manson gives a detailed account of a disease which he regarded as an affection peculiar to Europeans long resident in the tropics; he laid stress on the insidious onset, the tendency to relapse and the involvement of the tongue and mouth.

Van der Burg adopted the same designation " spruw," by which name a chronic diarrhoea had long been known in Java (*vide supra*), in an accurate clinical study in which, in all important points, he bore out Manson's description, save that he regarded the disease as being prevalent, but to a much less marked degree, amongst the native population.

In 1884 Maclean in his Lectures on the diseases of tropical climates, referred, apparently without knowledge of Manson's or Van der Burg's works, to the disease under the name of " scorbutic diarrhoea," and advised that it should be treated by anti-scorbutic measures.

Thin, who began writing on this subject in 1883, condensed much of the then existing knowledge and under the title of *Psilosis or Sprue* published a considerable volume in 1897. In this classical monograph he not only illustrated various sprue lesions of the tongue, but gave a very accurate description of the disease and its treatment by a milk and fruit diet, a line of treatment previously suggested by Manson in China and Van der Burg in Java.

Since that date various short articles on sprue have appeared which do not contribute very much to our knowledge of the subject, such as the papers on the pathology by Faber (1904), by Galloway (1905), by Richartz, and by Van der Scheer who considers a mild inflammation of the appendix to be the basis of the disorder. In 1906 there appeared a most valuable summary of our knowledge by Rademaker which supplies not only some original observations, but also gives an accurate account of the Dutch literature.

Finally Justi (1913, *Beiheft Archiv f. Schiffs- und Tropen-Hyg.* XVII, 1) gives a very full account of the microscopical findings in a case observed by him in Hong Kong.

In addition to the foregoing a number of short papers have appeared from time to time in the *Lancet* and *British Medical Journal* to which I shall refer in the sequel.

The latest, fullest and most accurate description of the disease in this or in any other language will be found in a monograph by Carnegie-Brown published in 1908.

A small volume by Begg (1912) deals chiefly with a form of treatment by santonin, a treatment which he claims has given good results.

Careful text-book accounts are to be found in Manson's *Tropical Diseases* (1914), and an article by the same writer in Allbutt and Rolleston's *System of Medicine* (1907), also in Scheube's *Die Krankheiten der Wärmer Länder* (1903), by Van der Scheer in Mense's *Handbuch der Tropenkrankheiten* (1909), and Daniels' *Tropical Medicine and Hygiene* (1912).

CHAPTER VIII

GENERAL GEOGRAPHICAL DISTRIBUTION OF SPRUE

SOME writers have asserted that sprue has a well-defined geographical distribution and that its home is essentially in the East, thereby suggesting some peculiar local cause. More recent evidence indicates that sprue has probably a world-wide tropical and subtropical distribution.

It is, I think, incontestable that Hillary's original description in 1766 referred to this disease in Barbados, but it is a noteworthy fact that since that date records of its occurrence in that island are singularly few. It may be that Hillary confounded sprue with pellagra, a disease in which the terminal symptoms are somewhat similar.

In a recent able and critical paper Ashford has described many undoubted cases of sprue occurring in Porto Rico. Undoubtedly the disease occurs with similar frequency in the other Antilles and probably throughout the whole American tropical zone. Such an inference is supported by cases reported from Haiti, Mexico and the north coast of S. America. As Ashford puts it, the circumstance that hitherto the chronic endemic diarrhoeas of these parts have not been designated sprue does not negative its previous existence there or justify the suggestion that sprue has disappeared from the West Indies and S. America subsequently to Hillary's time.

However, it is a fact that sprue is more frequently encountered in its most virulent form in Europeans hailing from the seaports of our Eastern possessions. Its apparent scarcity in some Eastern towns and its apparent prevalence in others may be ascribed in part to our inadequate knowledge of its aetiology and diagnosis.

It is so prevalent in Java that Van der Burg is stated to have seen no fewer than 1407 cases in Batavia alone.

In the French settlements of Tonquin and Annam sprue appears to be exceptionally prevalent. Undoubtedly it is the same disease as the "diarrhée de Cochin-Chine" which, as is well known, has decimated the European troops in these countries.

The paucity of records of sprue from Tropical Africa, considering the numbers of Europeans now visiting and resident in these parts, is a noteworthy fact. Begg, however, has reported cases from the Gold Coast, Upper Congo, and even from Morocco.

All evidence points to sprue being a regional as opposed to a climatic disease, seeing that it has been reported from places so climatically different as Java, Amoy, Shanghai and even from the temperate parts of Japan where the climate more nearly resembles that of Central Russia than that of the tropics.

It has been asserted, especially by Dutch authorities, that sprue originated in Sumatra and that it is extending its range. The evidence for this is not convincing.

One fact may be accepted as certain, that instances of genuine sprue arising *de novo* in permanent residents of temperate Europe are very rare and have seldom been recorded[1]. Cases such as those mentioned by Begg as originating in England must be looked upon with suspicion; sometimes they have proved to be instances of chronic pancreatitis, the symptoms of which in general resemble those of sprue.

Any statements about the absence of sprue in a given tropical or subtropical climate should be received with caution. The disease may really occur in places where it is reported to be absent. It may not have been recognised. Such evidence must be weighed with greater caution, in view of recent experience of pellagra and ankylostomiasis in this country and in the United States. This should lead to hesitation in making or accepting negative statements on such a point. In later years Thin recognised two types of sprue each having its special regional distribution. Though agreeing with him in the main, Carnegie-Brown points out that even now in many places most of the deaths it occasions are ascribed to other causes and that therefore estimates of its prevalence and severity based on unsatisfactory diagnosis are of little value.

The following is a list of localities from which sprue has been reported: India, Burma, Siam, Malay States, Straits Settlements, Cochin China, China, Japan, Java, Sumatra, Celebes, Macassar, Borneo, Ceylon, Philippines, N. Australia (Queensland), Fiji, Porto Rico, Haiti, West Indies, Mexico, S. America, Gold Coast, Upper Congo and Morocco.

[1] Van der Scheer, who has had a large experience of the disease and is an authority on the subject, has seen apparently a typical case in a gentleman of thirty-five years of age who had never been out of Holland. Mense in a private letter to Justi (1913, *Beiheft Archiv f. Schiffs- u. Tropen-Hyg.* XVII, 10) has diagnosed a case in an inhabitant of Cassel, Germany.

CHAPTER IX

DISTRIBUTION OF SPRUE IN EUROPEANS IN CEYLON

THE distribution of the European population in Ceylon is peculiar in that in the low-country it is mainly aggregated in the large towns such as Galle and Colombo, whereas in the up-country or tea districts of the Central Province it is very scattered. It is difficult to determine the incidence of sprue in Europeans in the Colony as no statistics of the number of affected Europeans have ever been kept, nor is this to be wondered at considering that all European are necessarily "private" cases. The investigator has therefore to rely on hearsay evidence for much of his information.

It is quite improbable that I interviewed during my visit every case of sprue in the European population. This much I can state that in the considerable number of sprue cases in Europeans about whom I obtained trustworthy information there was no striking disproportionate preponderance, if due allowance is made for certain circumstances, in the number of cases in which the disease originated at sea-level and those which originated at a higher elevation. Every effort was made to obtain accuracy in this part of the work. It is possible of course that in several or all of the high country cases the infection was acquired in the low-country. Against such a supposition is the fact that the high country tea planters generally reside in their own districts for a great number of years consecutively and, as I discovered in several specific instances, seldom visit the low-country and then only for very short periods. The resident European population of Colombo and that of the elevated Central Province are about equal in number (Appendix II). Bearing this in mind a reference to the map (Text-fig. 1) will convince the reader that there is at least no marked disproportion between the low and the elevated districts as regards the liability of Europeans to sprue in Ceylon. There are practically no European residents in any town north of Colombo and but very few on the East Coast in towns such as Trincomalee and Batticaloa; this explains the absence of sprue in these parts as indicated by the map.

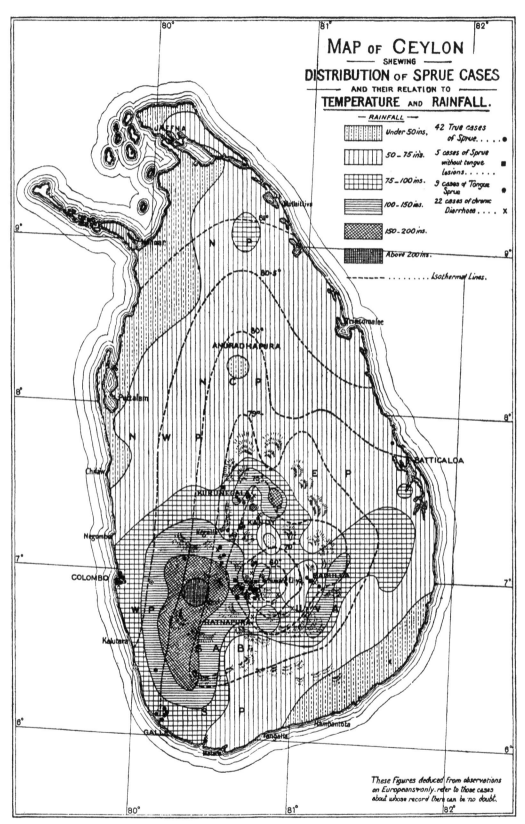

MAP OF CEYLON
SHEWING
DISTRIBUTION OF SPRUE CASES
AND THEIR RELATION TO
TEMPERATURE AND RAINFALL.

— RAINFALL —

	Under 50 ins.	42 True cases of Sprue..... ●
	50 - 75 ins.	5 cases of Sprue without tongue lesions..... ■
	75 - 100 ins.	9 cases of Tongue Sprue..... ●
	100 - 150 ins.	22 cases of chronic Diarrhœa X
	150 - 200 ins.	
	Above 200 ins.	

.... Isothermal Lines.

These figures deduced from observations
on Europeans only, refer to those cases
about whose record there can be no doubt.

B. S.   Fig. 1   2

The influence of climate on the incidence of the disease. I must refer the reader to the paragraph on the geographical distribution of the disease on page 14, where evidence is given of the occurrence of sprue in subtropical climates such as Japan, thereby suggesting that distribution is not dependent on climate alone; even in the tropics it apparently bears no invariable relation to atmospheric conditions— temperature, moisture, etc. An authentic case, leading to a fatal result, occurred in a lady resident since childhood in Nuwara Eliya, a town where the average mean temperature is 58° F., or 22° F. lower than that of Colombo (Appendix III). It is also apparent from the map referred to that the distribution of the disease is not connected with the amount of rainfall.

Out of 28 cases of sprue in Europeans which I personally investigated

12	apparently	contracted	the disease	in	the low country
2	,,	,,	,,	between	1000–2000 ft.
3	,,	,,	,,	,,	2000–3000 ft.
3	,,	,,	,,	,,	3000–4000 ft.
6	,,	,,	,,	,,	4000–5000 ft.
1	,,	,,	,,	at	5000 ft.
1	,,	,,	,,	,,	6000 ft.

The European population of the Southern and Western Provinces is 3557 as against 2679 in the Central Province. On reference to the map, records of 13 cases in the Southern and Western and of 28 cases in the Central Provinces will be found. These figures appear to be in direct contradiction to the statement I have already made; but it must be borne in mind that the Europeans in the hot and damp Southern and Western Provinces cannot, by any means, be considered as residents in the same sense as the planters in the Central Province. The usual term of residence in the low-country for Europeans, whether engaged in commerce or planting, is three years, while the planters and other Europeans in the temperate climate of the Central Province are often resident continuously for ten years or longer, and one would think that, in consequence of this prolonged residence, the incidence of the disease amongst the latter would necessarily be greater.

CHAPTER X

CERTAIN FACTORS IN THEIR BEARING ON THE INCIDENCE OF SPRUE

(1) *Race in its bearing on the liability to sprue*

(a) *The occurrence of sprue in native races.* All writers are in agreement on one point, namely, that sprue is preeminently a disease of the European in the tropics and that the native is only occasionally, if ever, affected.

Some, notably Manson, have recorded that, in their experience, no case in a pure blooded native has ever come under their observation.

Van der Burg evidently recognised the disease in Javanese, Malays, Papuans, Negroes and Arabs, but considered the lighter coloured Chinese more frequently attacked than the darker skinned races, and then only after a long period of residence in the endemic area. He only saw 32 native cases during a thirty years residence in Java. Van der Scheer concluded that as compared with the white the dark races were by 30 per cent. less liable to the disease. Buchanan considered sprue to be identical with the " famine diarrhoea " so frequently encountered in the poorer natives of India. Graham has noted the disease in natives of Sumatra, but states that all forms of stomatitis are called sprue by them, in this manner leading to great confusion. Galloway records that sprue occurs, but is uncommon in the inhabitants of Java, Sumatra, Philippines, Cochin-China and Straits Settlements, and in a series of 87 cases observed by him native cases formed 37 per cent. of the whole. Jefferys and Maxwell in their *Diseases of China* (1910) mention a typical case in a Chinawoman. Ashworth (1913) has recognised the disease in natives of Porto Rico and the Antilles. Discounting all extraneous factors, I am convinced that sprue in native races is of much more common occurrence than has been supposed hitherto. There are certain real difficulties in recognising in an Eastern native a disease of such an ill-defined nature as sprue; these difficulties I have been able fully to appreciate during the course of my researches.

2—2

In dealing with the ignorant native one must emphasise firstly, that no details of personal history can be obtained or, if obtained, relied upon. In making a diagnosis the investigator has, therefore, to depend upon physical signs alone and these, it must be confessed, are often indefinite enough. Secondly, it is a matter of common knowledge that the stools of natives, subsisting as they do for the most part on farinaceous food, rice as a rule, are lighter coloured, more bulky and of a looser consistency than those of the European. Furthermore, caste prejudice militates against the systematic examination of the excreta. Thirdly, the common habit of betel-chewing, by staining the buccal mucosa, tends to disguise its condition; and fourthly the common occurrence in natives of various forms of stomatitis makes a diagnosis of sprue from the mouth symptoms an extremely difficult matter. Fifthly, anaemia, caused by ankylostome infection and by the malaria parasite, is of such frequent occurrence amongst them as to still further complicate the matter. Each and all of these factors must be discounted before one is justified in diagnosing sprue in a native.

DESCRIPTION OF PLATE I

Fig. 1. Sprue tongue in a native case.

Fig. 2. Smooth atrophic tongue of chronic ankylostomiasis.

Fig. 3. First appearance of sprue inflammation on tongue.

Fig. 4. A smooth area on tongue resulting from previous sprue inflammation.

Fig. 5. Appearance of tongue two years after apparent recovery from sprue.

Fig. 6. A haemorrhage into a fungiform papilla on chronic sprue tongue.

Fig. 7. Sprue tongue, chronic stage.

Fig. 8. Sprue tongue, acute stage. Death three weeks later.

Fig. 9. Appearance of thrush on sprue tongue; native case, immediately before death.

Fig. 10. Sprue tongue three weeks before death. A very anaemic case; *vide* text, post-mortem B.

Fig. 11. Aphthous ulcer on sprue tongue.

Fig. 12. Sprue tongue. Appearance before treatment.

Fig. 13. Hypertrophy of fungiform papillae in a normal native.

Fig. 14. Sprue tongue showing regeneration of papillae. Appearance after $4\frac{1}{2}$ months treatment (same case as shown in Fig. 12).

Fig. 15. Completely denuded tongue, an extreme degree of "Tongue Sprue" in a Sinhalese prisoner.

Fig. 16. Tongue sprue in a male European.

Fig. 17. The leucomatous tongue found generally in association with stomatitis in natives.

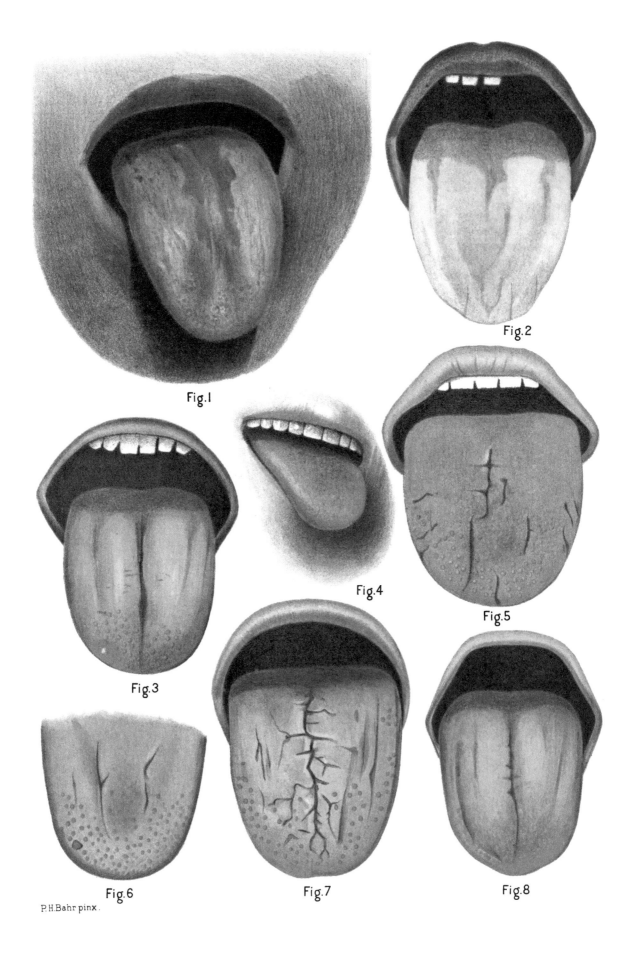

Fig.1

Fig.2

Fig.3

Fig.4

Fig.5

Fig.6

Fig.7

Fig.8

P.H.Bahr pinx.

PLATE I

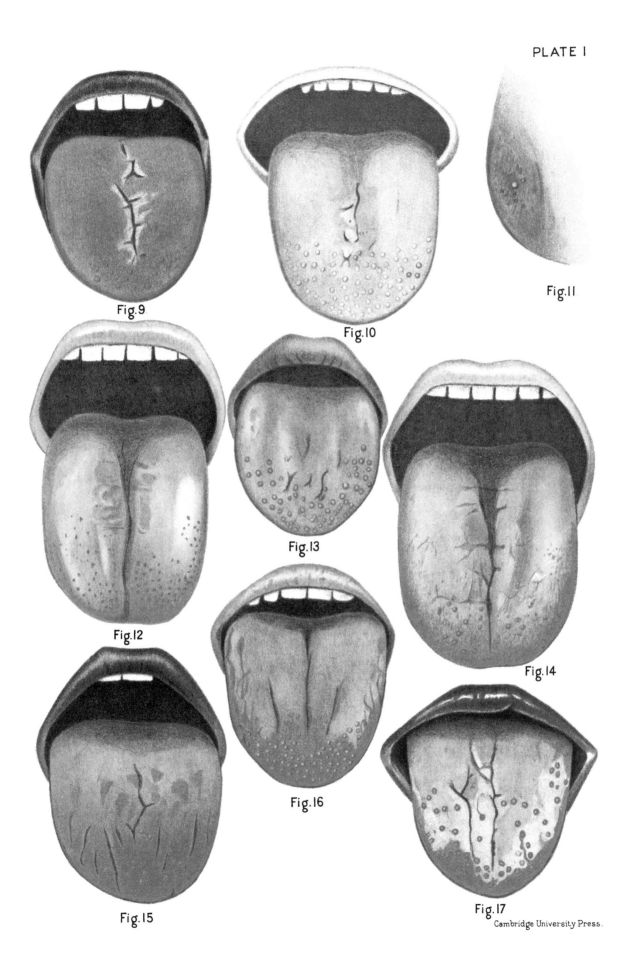

Fig.9

Fig.10

Fig.11

Fig.12

Fig.13

Fig.14

Fig.15

Fig.16

Fig.17

Cambridge University Press.

I have collected notes of eleven cases occurring in natives about the diagnosis of which there can be little doubt. On referring to Appendix IV, where short notes of each case are given, the reader will gather that the disease occurred in my experience in members of several races, in Moors, Sinhalese, Indians, as well as in the country-bred Tamil coolie. As five of my native cases were seen shortly before death and tissues secured from three post-mortems, although in only one was a complete examination permitted, the diagnosis may be relied upon.

In these eleven native cases, all males, the tongue was smooth and devoid of papillae, and in four cases which rapidly proved fatal, it was covered by a slimy growth of the thrush fungus. In combination with the typical tongue, the other cardinal sprue symptoms—such as constant diarrhoea, great anaemia and abdominal distension—were present. My difficulties in arriving at a positive diagnosis of sprue in some of these cases during life was increased by the presence of ankylostome ova in the stools of five, and in one case in addition to these ova, of the vegetative and cystic forms of *Entamoeba coli* and *Trichomonas intestinalis*. Besides these eleven male cases a number of diarrhoea cases in women, of apparently the same nature, but which for various reasons could not be thoroughly investigated, were seen in the wards of the Lady Havelock Hospital in Colombo.

In searching through a native hospital it is a common event to find amongst the diarrhoea cases of various natures and origin one or more cases differing from the others in general external appearance, in the bare tongue, distended abdomen, earthy complexion and oedematous extremities (Plate I, fig. 1). In the majority of such cases it is impossible to say whether the clinical picture is the result of primary uncomplicated sprue, or of ankylostomiasis, or of sprue with a superimposed ankylostome[1] infection. Failing to find ankylostome ova in the stools of a case presenting these symptoms, I considered myself justified in regarding it as a genuine case of sprue.

It is difficult to ascertain whether these bare tongues cause the patient discomfort. The uneducated natives are prone, regardless of

---

[1] It is probable that every native harbours ankylostomes though usually in numbers too small to cause any symptoms. One must bear in mind that a negative microscopical examination, as usually made, of the stools does not preclude such an infection. According to Boycott and Bruns (1911, *Lancet*, I, 786), only 40 per cent. of the cases can be diagnosed by direct microscopical examination, 55 per cent. by Bass' gravitation method, but 99 per cent. by a method of artificially cultivating the larvae from ova.

the accuracy of the statement, to reply to questions in a sense which, in their opinion, the interrogator desires or expects. Aversion to their favourite pungent curries may be taken as an indication of sensitiveness of the buccal mucous membrane and is a safer method of ascertaining the truth than any statement they may make.

(b) *Sprue in Burghers.* Among the educated Burghers eight typical cases of sprue were seen, none of these had any ankylostome infection, although three had ova of *Trichocephalus dispar* in their stools. These were all typical cases and there was no doubt about the diagnosis. I shall have occasion frequently to refer to them later.

(c) *Sprue in Europeans.* Cases of sprue were seen in 36 Europeans, five of whom were born in Ceylon and had never left the Colony.

It will be gathered from these figures that all the races represented in Ceylon are liable to the disease and further that the immigrant European is probably particularly liable to contract the infection. The latter supposition is strengthened by the relatively small number of cases seen in the Burgher as compared with the immigrant European community, although the former is at least three times as numerous as the latter.

(2) *Incubation period*

The limits of this are difficult to ascertain. Galloway cites a case in which the disease developed after only a ten months residence in Malaya, and Roux gives other instances of its occurrence in Europeans who had contracted the disease on their first visit to the tropics and after but a twenty-four hours stay in an Eastern port; such cases, however, must be of great rarity.

Duration of residence. In the series of cases in Europeans studied by me in Ceylon, the average duration of residence in the island or eastern tropics before symptoms of sprue commenced was about twenty years. The shortest periods of which I have accurate records were six weeks and three months respectively after landing in Ceylon.

(3) *Special liability of the female sex*

Of my thirty-six cases of sprue in Europeans nineteen were females and only seventeen males. These figures bear out the opinion generally held that the female sex is specially susceptible to the disease. The preponderating liability of the female is evident if we remember that in Ceylon the proportion of European males to females is almost two to one. According to the last census there were 4600 male to 2900 female Europeans resident in the island.

(4) *Age*

It is generally stated that sprue is seldom seen in Europeans below middle age or in those long resident in the endemic area. Nevertheless it may develop at any age even in children of European parentage.

Van der Burg states that he has recognised the disease in children of one and a half to four years of age, though it is as a general rule extremely rare in young adults. The oldest man I saw in Ceylon suffering from sprue symptoms, was a Burgher of seventy-six years of age; the oldest European, a man of seventy; the youngest was a boy of thirteen of mixed parentage. I have, however, reason to believe that the disease occurs in natives at a still earlier age. I saw a Tamil boy of eight who presented typical sprue symptoms, of which he died four months later.

(5) *Occupation*

That the disease is not limited to any particular occupation or industry is patent to anyone who has seriously considered the subject. Out of a series of forty-six typical cases, twenty-one, or the greater number, were planters who form the bulk of the European population; others were Government clerks, engineers, a station master, a missionary, shop-assistants, a postmaster, a smelter, a proctor, a merchant and a needle-woman.

Out of twenty cases of chronic diarrhoea, but without tongue lesions, fifteen were planters, the rest were store-keepers, school teachers, etc.

(6) *The influence of housing*

At the present day and as a general rule Europeans on tea and rubber plantations are comfortably housed. The site selected for the bungalow is generally the highest and most open part of the estate, if possible in the vicinity of a jungle stream from which a water supply may be obtained.

The majority of the houses are single storied, roomy, wooden buildings, with a tile or shingle roof. On a large estate there are several such bungalows for the accommodation of the superintendent and his assistants. The coolie lines and cattle sheds are usually separated by a distance of about a quarter of a mile from the European quarters. The estate superintendent spends a considerable part of his time in his tea or rubber factory, a large building situated some distance from the bungalow and generally in the vicinity of a stream supplying water power. At the present day the older wooden European bungalows and factories are generally giving way to more modern structures of brick and stone.

"*Dry-rot.*" There is a popular and prevalent idea amongst the planting community of Ceylon that sprue originates solely in bungalows attacked with dry-rot. Such houses are notoriously unhealthy. Dr Drummond of Talawakelle, as a result of personal observation, was led to believe that the unhealthiness of the estate bungalows in Ceylon was a most important factor in predisposing to sprue. From the rotten condition of the timbers the planters have designated such houses "dry-rot bungalows." The dry-rot itself is a yellow sawdust-like powder and is commonly found in the centre of the affected timbers, especially those forming the roof, corner posts and the floor joists. The bungalows affected in this manner are generally thirty or more years old dating from the coffee-planting days, and were originally built with green, unseasoned timber; in these a yellow dust, emitting a peculiarly disagreeable smell, can commonly be seen in all the rooms into which it has fallen from the roof. As the basement floor is built flush with the ground and there is no subsoil drainage, the undersurface of the floor-boarding is frequently also in a rotten state. These rotten bungalows are found especially in the planting districts situated above the 3000 ft. level, seldom below that elevation. The explanation of this limitation as regards elevation appears to be that the sodden wood is liable to be attacked and often completely destroyed by white ants, an insect pest which does not occur at higher elevations. These insects form burrows which they line with red earth in the timber. It may be added that timber affected with the so-called "dry-rot" often appears to be perfectly sound when viewed from the outside, but on closer examination, it will be found to be riddled with weevil (*Curculionidae*) burrows. I was able to isolate from the crumbling timbers fungi of the genera *Penicillium*, *Aspergillus* and *Mucor*. Probably these moulds attack and soften the wood to such an extent that it is subsequently invaded by weevils, woodlice and other insects[1], thus leading to further disintegration and giving rise to a characteristic yellow dust.

As far as I could gather, the symptoms experienced by the inhabitants of such bungalows were just those most prone to arise from inhalation

---

[1] In addition to the white ant the following insects were found in the rotten wood: weevils (*Curculionidae*), woodlice (*Isopoda*), fish-insects (*Thysanura*), and some pupal cases and eggs of other unknown insects.

of this dust, which irritates the nasal passages and gives rise to sore throats and secretion of much ropy mucus, often combined with a feeling of lassitude, headaches, and seemingly in some instances of slight attacks of diarrhoea. The unhealthiness of some of these bungalows is so apparent and notorious that on account of it a succession of estate superintendents have been forced to quit their employment.

I was able to find only two such " dry-rot " bungalows in which more than one authentic case of sprue had occurred in recent years. In one of these I was able to see the present resident and his predecessor, both of whom were slightly affected. In the other instance three cases of pronounced sprue occurred at long intervals.

I personally visited the localities in which twenty-six Europeans and Burghers first developed symptoms of the disease; twelve originated in well-known dry-rot bungalows; seven in new wooden buildings where the suspicion of dry-rot could not be entertained, six in stone houses, two in mud houses, two in a modern hotel in Colombo; one in a monastery, one on board ship, and one on a canal boat. Additional information was obtained through the kindness of the Planters' Association which distributed to over 1700 estates printed forms containing questions amongst other things bearing on this particular point; 143 of these circulars were returned to me carefully filled in, the results of which I have summarised in Appendix V. From this it can be seen that these " dry-rot " bungalows are generally of great age, that they are mostly on tea estates and that a certain number of sprue cases have originated in them from time to time.

It cannot be affirmed that the evidence I have collected establishes or justifies the popular idea that " dry-rot " is directly connected with sprue, but, just as any unhealthy environment would do, it may predispose to development of this disease by reducing the normal vital resistance.

(7) *Water supply in relation to sprue*

On most of the Ceylon plantations, especially on those supervised by Europeans, great care is taken to secure a pure water supply. The stream sources supplying the bungalows are jealously guarded and are in some instances covered in. The drinking water is almost invariably boiled before use, and on the evidence collected, I conclude that as a medium of sprue infection water might be dismissed. Of the sprue cases in which special enquiries were made, sixteen were in the habit of drinking the town water, eleven spring, five well, two rain water, while one had drunk only soda water since his arrival in the Colony.

(8) *The influence of food and sanitation*

From the fact that sprue occurs in all races frequenting or inhabiting Ceylon, each race living on its special diet, it is improbable that food plays any part in the aetiology of this disease. Since curry has been incriminated by certain writers, I deemed it advisable to address enquiries to twenty-nine Europeans suffering from sprue with regard to this special article of food and learned that five of them had never partaken of curries or other highly flavoured spices during their residence in the island.

In all European houses in Ceylon, with the exception of the more modern ones in Colombo, dry earth closets are still in vogue. These are generally cleaned out twice daily. Night soil disposal therefore plays little if any part in the production of sprue. Cases originate in the best Colombo hotels, which are provided with water-drainage and every similar modern convenience.

(9) *Possibility of an insect conveyer*

Considerable attention has been given to this point. Only a few species of mosquito are common both to the low-country and to the hill-country. Only three species of *Anopheles* and three species of *Culex* were captured above 2500 ft. In Appendix VI will be found a list of those collected in different parts of the island. These insects are neither numerous nor troublesome in any place above 2500 ft.

I could obtain no evidence of the presence of other biting insects, such as *Simulidae*, in any of the up-country streams, though they have been reported from Kandy. *Phlebotomus*, or the sand fly, is common only in the hot dry areas such as Anuradhapura and Trincomalee. There is, of course, a possibility that sprue is carried by a non-biting fly or other insect such as *Musca domestica*. The last-named has a curious distribution in Ceylon; it is much more in evidence in the tea districts, where the decomposing tea refuse affords it suitable breeding places, than it is in the low-country.

(10) *Previous disease considered as a predisposing cause*

The development of some chronic infection or some debilitating disease is regarded as the most potent of all the causes predisposing to sprue, and of these the most important is undoubtedly dysentery. Every writer on the subject has remarked on this fact; Manson has described "sprue secondary to dysentery" as a distinct variety of the disease; Carnegie-Brown has also laid special stress on this point. Some have gone so far as to suggest that the condition known as sprue is actually the ultimate result of chronic dysentery itself; by others it has been considered that the development of the sprue organism, whatever may be its nature, in the intestinal canal is favoured by frequent dysenteric attacks.

Amongst my series of cases the occurrence of previous dysenteric attacks is a noticeable feature, but it is open to doubt whether these are not merely coincidental, seeing that the majority of European residents have, at one time or other, been subject to such attacks. Out of fifty-five cases of sprue in Europeans and Burghers, about whom I have accurate information on the point, in seventeen the sprue symptoms supervened after an attack of dysentery. In half of this number the dysentery occurred four or more years previously. In seven females the symptoms set in soon after confinement. In two (one male and one female) they supervened on hill diarrhoea contracted in India, in two (males) after syphilis and lastly in one (male) symptoms developed after an accident resulting in the loss of one arm.

In nearly half my cases the disease arose without evident pre-disposing cause. I think, therefore, there are ample grounds for regarding sprue as a primary specific infection, but that, like all other chronic infections, such as tuberculosis, any debilitating cause such as disease, physical exhaustion or unhealthy surroundings by lowering the vital resistance may render the alimentary tract more liable to attack by the specific sprue germ.

CHAPTER XI

SPRUE REGARDED AS AN INFECTIOUS DISEASE

THE occurrence of sprue in Ceylon in all classes of the community irrespective of age, sex, race, diet, occupation and conditions of environment suggests an infection and the communicability of the disease from man to man.

The contagion-theory of sprue has already been advanced by Galloway (1905, *Journ. Trop. Med.* 289, and *Brit. Med. Journ.* II, 1284). This author has cited native and Eurasian cases occurring in husband and wife, father and daughter and mother and daughter; furthermore, he has noted the development of the symptoms in a lady five years after her marriage to a man who had temporarily recovered from sprue.

In my short experience in Ceylon occurrences of this nature were far too frequent to be purely accidental. Thus:

(1) A Eurasian woman who had typical symptoms—aphthae, sore tongue and diarrhoea—died in April 1912. Up to the last stages of the disease she was in the habit of feeding her youngest son, a boy of thirteen and her constant companion, with portions of her food and with the spoon she herself used. In November 1911, this boy developed a sore tongue and diarrhoea, and when I saw him, in June 1912, he presented all the appearances of a typical case of sprue.

(2) An elderly European gentleman, over fifty years resident in Ceylon, developed sprue in 1901, while living with his sister. The latter developed the disease and eventually died of it. The gentleman's married daughter while residing in the same house contracted a chronic diarrhoea from which she was still intermittently suffering when I saw her in 1912.

(3) Through the courtesy of Dr Cantlie I have been able to follow out an instance of the disease occurring in husband and wife. In 1893 a Ceylon tea planter developed symptoms from which he eventually

died in 1898. Two years after, while resident in England, his widow became ill with identically the same symptoms.

(4) A planter contracted sprue in 1908, a year after he had left Ceylon, and died in England apparently of its effects in May 1913. An elderly single lady living in the same bungalow with him also commenced to suffer from symptoms before he left the country, and was treated subsequently in England. When I saw her in February 1913 she was suffering from a severe relapse.

(5) An old Irish lady, long resident in Colombo, had been suffering from symptoms for about four months. A fortnight before I saw this lady her daughter, with whom she lived, had developed diarrhoea and tongue symptoms which were well marked at the time of my examination.

(6) I treated a lady, a planter's wife, for a typical relapse of sprue. A young planter living in the same house with this patient consulted me on account of a chronic diarrhoea for which he had eventually to return to Europe and which he had contracted shortly after his arrival in Ceylon.

(In addition to these cases, instances came to my notice in which children born of sprue-infected mothers suffered for a long time from chronic diarrhoea which in one at least to my knowledge proved fatal.)

It may be that the occurrence of the disease in people, so closely associated with one another as in the foregoing instances, is merely coincidental; but I am inclined to believe the evidence is in favour of direct infection by a specific, but as a rule avirulent, organism. The long incubation period and the prolonged latency which this disease exhibits suggest feebleness of pathogenic power in the hypothetical germ and the importance of predisposing influences for the development of the disease.

All my attempts to communicate sprue to the lower animals failed. The animals experimented with were guineapigs and monkeys (*Macacus*). It is possible that the experiments were not on an extensive enough scale or that only the higher apes are liable to this infection.

The following is a short summary of my experiments:

(1) *With saliva and scrapings from sprue tongues.*

A. A monkey was anaesthetised and inoculated on the inner surface of the cheek with material derived from an inflamed sprue tongue. The monkey died a week after of diarrhoea, which was probably in no way related to sprue seeing that two non-inoculated control animals died of diarrhoea also at the same time.

B.   5 c.c. of sprue saliva were introduced by means of a catheter into the stomach of an anaesthetised monkey.   Though this animal was kept under observation for a period of six months no symptoms of any sort developed.

C.   A guineapig was inoculated intraperitoneally with 2 c.c. of sprue saliva. It remained in perfect health.

(2)   *With sprue stools.*

A.   A monkey was anaesthetised and 30 c.c. of a watery extract of a sprue stool introduced by means of a catheter into the alimentary canal; half was injected into the stomach and the remainder into the rectum.   No ill effects of any sort were subsequently noted.

B.   A guineapig injected intraperitoneally with 2 c.c. of a similar extract remained subsequently in perfect health.

CHAPTER XII

SYMPTOMS OF SPRUE AS MET WITH IN CEYLON

THE material for the study of symptoms and of clinical histories of sprue was obtained from Europeans and educated Burghers who could be relied upon to give an accurate and intelligible account of their illnesses. I need hardly say that the symptoms of the disease and its manifestations varied very considerably. As a result of my study, I conclude that Manson's classification founded on a clinical basis is the only one which can afford any satisfaction. It is a classification which rests on the hypothesis that the disease process, whatever that may be, affects the several regions of the intestinal canal to an unequal degree, thus giving rise to symptoms varying according to the region of the alimentary canal more specially involved.

Under the heading of *complete or typical sprue* I include all cases exhibiting the two cardinal symptoms—the characteristic tongue and the typical stools. This category includes cases of all degrees of severity suggesting therefore a further subdivision into mild, acute and chronic.

Under the heading of *incomplete sprue* I include a number of cases in which, though the typical diarrhoea was present, no pathological changes of the tongue or of the buccal mucous membranes could be distinguished. I have felt obliged to include under this heading a large series of diarrhoeas (mostly occurring in young male Europeans) of an explosive nature accompanied by emaciation, flatulence and dyspepsia, and which, in the absence of any better explanation, I am inclined to regard as early cases of intestinal sprue. I will discuss later on the possibility of these cases being of the same nature as hill diarrhoea.

As a further subdivision of incomplete sprue I include under the designation "*tongue sprue*" cases in which, though the mouth symptoms and tongue changes were present, yet the disease process did not appear to have spread beyond the buccal cavity. That sprue may be limited to the buccal cavity has not, as far as I can gather, been previously noted. Although some such classification is desirable it must not be on hard and fast lines. There are cases recorded in my note-books in which one type merges imperceptibly into another.

A.   Typical or complete sprue

It is unnecessary to give in detail the clinical histories of all my cases. I have, therefore, compressed the mass of information collected into as short a space as is possible.

The earliest symptoms noted varied widely in different patients, in the majority the onset of the disease was an insidious one. In only four instances could I elicit a history of an initial acute diarrhoea, merging later into a more chronic form. In eleven cases, on the other hand, tongue symptoms (in two persisting for as long as three years before the commencement of the diarrhoea) were the only indications of the onset of the disease. In five, the onset of the diarrhoea and the tongue symptoms concurred.

The group can be further subdivided under four headings:

Subgroup 1. Cases with both marked tongue and diarrhoea symptoms.

Subgroup 2. Cases with acute diarrhoea and subacute tongue symptoms.

Subgroup 3. Cases with subacute tongue and mild diarrhoea symptoms.

Subgroup 4. Chronic cases.

Subgroup 1. *Cases with both marked tongue and diarrhoea symptoms*

Eleven clinical cases, three females and eight males, could be included under this heading. In three instances no aphthae were ever seen in the mouth, though the tongue symptoms were marked during the whole time the patients remained under my observation; nor could a history of any buccal ulceration be obtained, a fact of importance from an aetiological standpoint. The inflammation of the tongue was accompanied in many instances by loss of taste sense and excessive salivation. A history of dysphagia could be obtained only in two in whom the tongue symptoms were also very acute. Acute dyspepsia, relieved by frequent vomiting, was also a dominating symptom in these two cases[1]. All the eleven patients complained of flatulent distension of the lower part of the abdomen, causing a degree of discomfort which increased towards the later hours of the day and was

---

[1] I saw two cases in which the gastric symptoms so dominated the clinical picture that they might with justice be termed "gastric sprue." So far as could be ascertained by combined auscultation and percussion a definite dilatation of the stomach was associated with these symptoms.

only temporarily relieved by the passage of stool, accompanied by a sense of exhaustion.

A curious point, and one noted by Carnegie-Brown and others, was the apparent periodicity and alternation of the symptoms, the amelioration of the mouth symptoms during an attack of diarrhoea, and *vice versa*. A history was frequently given of rectal irritation, especially after such an attack of diarrhoea, but no aphthous ulceration of the anal orifice was ever observed. Progressive emaciation was noted in every case, even in one lady in whom, though the stools were bulky and the mouth and tongue symptoms very acute, diarrhoea was absent. The amount of emaciation in any individual patient appeared to be proportionate to the length of time the illness had lasted. In several cases a loss of three stone or more in a period of five to six months was recorded. The exacerbation of symptoms resulting from any physical or mental strain was most noticeable, especially in women during pregnancy and after child-birth.

Pigmentation[1] (or excessive freckling), twice on the temple and once in axilla, and consisting of brown patches of irregular outline, was noted in three anaemic cases.

In none could I elicit by percussion any marked diminution of the liver dulness. No cardiac derangement, save a certain amount of blurring of the first sound, was noted.

Subgroup 2. *Cases with acute diarrhoea and subacute tongue symptoms*

In this category I have placed a series of twenty-two cases, eleven occurring in women and the remainder in men. In these the illness ran a much more rapid course than in those included under the first heading. In two of these cases I was able to make a thorough post-mortem examination.

In none of these twenty-two cases were the tongue changes of a marked character. They consisted solely of inflammation of the tip and sides of the organ, a condition which inconvenienced the patient only when partaking of highly spiced or very hot food, in fact two of the male patients only realised any inconvenience when smoking

---

[1] Abnormalities of pigmentation are of common occurrence in the intestinal toxaemias. This abnormal dark brown pigment is of a similar nature to that of haemochromatosis; it is apparently not produced by urobilin, but more probably by an admixture of haemosiderin, and an iron free pigment haemofuscin. Ledingham (1913, *Proc. Roy. Soc. Med.* VI. (supp.), 153).

strong pipe-tobacco, an occurrence which first drew attention to the appearance of their tongues.

In six instances the tongue symptoms were noted before the onset of the diarrhoea. In three they were of so mild a character as to cause the patient no great inconvenience, as far as could be ascertained, during the whole course of the illness which ultimately terminated fatally.

It is important to note the absence of a history of buccal aphthae in four instances of this type (Subgroup 2) of case. Two of these were observed daily during the terminal stages of their illness. In one the onset of sprue was secondary to an attack of what was diagnosed as hill diarrhoea contracted in Ootacamund in Southern India.

In seven advanced and anaemic cases, curious pigmentations of the skin were noted consisting of dark brown patches of irregular outline resembling exaggerated freckles, situated in four cases on the forehead (Plate II, fig. 1), temple and cheek, in two cases on the abdomen and in the seventh case on the legs. Apparently this form of pigmentation is dependent on the intense anaemia as the patches disappeared after treatment, and directly an improvement in the general condition of the patient set in.

From a detailed examination of fourteen of these cases in an advanced stage of the disease (in two instances a few weeks before death) I was unable to make out by percussion the diminution of the liver dulness on which so much stress has been laid by some writers; in five only was I able to demonstrate any appreciable diminution, but nothing suggesting a shrinkage comparable to that in acute atrophy of the liver.

In the majority of cases no abnormality could be detected by a physical examination of the heart; but in three advanced cases a basal systolic murmur, of probable haemic origin, was noted. In a fourth a presystolic mitral murmur indicated a stenosis, probably of a rheumatic origin.

Of great interest is one particular case in whom the first symptoms of the disease were noted after seven years residence in England[1]. This patient was a very corpulent man, weighing over 280 lbs. He lost 84 lbs. during the course of his illness lasting over a year; his recovery was apparently complete, and he has now resided in Ceylon for the last eight years without any further recurrence of symptoms.

---

[1] Thin has recorded a similar case in a man who developed symptoms of sprue seventeen years after his return to Europe.

PLATE II

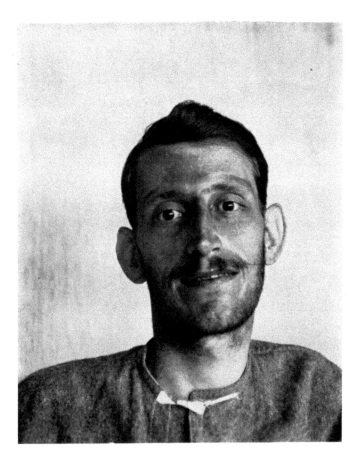

Fig. 1. Case of sprue showing pigmentation of forehead. Photograph by the Author.

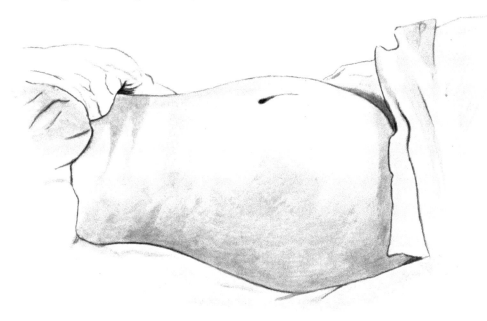

Fig. 2. Case of sprue showing characteristic meteorism, tongue symptoms being absent.
Drawing by the Author.

(Both of these figures are reproduced by kind permission of the Society of Tropical Medicine and Hygiene.)

Subgroup 3. *Cases with subacute tongue and mild diarrhoea symptoms*

In this category I have included a series of twelve cases, eight in women and four in men, all of whom are still resident in Ceylon and in good health. Their illness must have been of a very mild nature, as all symptoms disappeared after a short course of treatment or after a voyage to Europe. In none could the diarrhoea be termed acute. As a rule the patients gave a history of passing two or three large clay-coloured and sometimes frothy stools of a porridgy consistency in the early hours of the morning. A simultaneous onset of tongue and bowel symptoms was noted in three cases. In five instances the soreness of the tongue drew attention to the impending illness at some considerable period prior to the onset of the diarrhoea. Aphthae were seen, or a history of their occurrence was obtained, in eight out of the twelve cases.

Neither anaemia nor emaciation was a marked feature in any case. No abnormality, save perhaps a slight prominence and distension of the lower abdomen, was made out on clinical examination.

Subgroup 4. *Chronic sprue cases*

I have notes of two cases of chronic diarrhoea. Both were men over middle age and of over thirty years residence in the country. They gave a history of a prolonged subacute diarrhoea, generally occurring at night time or in the early hours of the morning. From time to time a spell of a more acute nature would supervene. In both cases the illness had been of long standing and accompanied by progressive emaciation. The stools were of a peculiar grey colour, porridgy in consistency, and becoming paler on a milk diet. In both cases I was able to detect by percussion an appreciable diminution in the liver dulness, and a distension of the lower abdomen, but in neither was there any history of aphthous ulceration of the mouth. The tongue was interesting, and was red, inflamed and superficially fissured both in a longitudinal and transverse direction; of the papillae the filiform had been completely destroyed, the fungiform being represented by a few prominent and highly polished remains (Plate I, fig. 7). Anaemia was not pronounced; the haemoglobin was about 75 per cent. of the normal and the red cells were reduced to about 3,000,000 per cm.

I wish to emphasise the apparently late involvement of the tongue; although considerable denudation had taken place, it appeared to cause the patients very little inconvenience. I am inclined to regard these cases as sprue in which the affection of the tongue and of the intestinal canal was of a very chronic nature.

B. INCOMPLETE SPRUE

I have given already a brief definition of what I mean by the term
"*incomplete sprue*." According to my experience in Ceylon, this
group may be subdivided on clinical grounds as follows:

(1) *Intestinal sprue.* Cases with typical *pale* stools and intestinal
symptoms, but with no involvement whatsoever of the tongue or mouth.

(2) Cases of chronic diarrhoea with *bilious*, frothy stools and other
sprue-like symptoms.

(3) *Tongue sprue.* Cases in which the disease is apparently limited
to the buccal cavity.

About the existence of the first subgroup there can be little doubt,
cases of this description have been recognised by Manson and other
authorities as being of the same nature as true sprue.

I am not so certain about the validity of the second and third
subgroups, but I will bring forward evidence pointing to the probability
that the underlying morbid process in them is of the same nature as
in ordinary sprue.

Subgroup 1. *Intestinal sprue without tongue symptoms*

Seven cases, four in men and three in women, were encountered.
The stools were typically clay coloured and frothy, but in no single
instance could any abnormal appearance of the tongue be detected,
although two cases gave a positive history of buccal aphthae. A history
of early morning diarrhoea, of a markedly cyclical character and
accompanied by vomiting and acute dyspepsia, was obtained in two of
the seven patients. In a third in whom the disease had lasted nearly
twelve years the atrophy and distension of the intestinal tract were
very marked as shown in Plate II, fig. 2; nevertheless no appreciable
diminution of the liver dulness could be detected by percussion and
the patient was not anaemic. In fact anaemia was not a marked
feature of any of these cases; and in no instance was a lower haemoglobin percentage than 80 recorded. Considerable emaciation, but not
to such a marked degree as in typical examples of the disease, was
noted in every one of the seven.

It may be argued that these are simply cases of chronic hill diarrhoea.
I think that in favour of this supposition only a small amount of evidence
can be adduced. The illness originated in all seven cases in different
localities and at different altitudes; in four cases the illness commenced
in Colombo or in the hot plains of the low-country, in the remaining
three at an elevation of above 3000 ft.

Subgroup 2. *Chronic diarrhoea with bilious frothy stools*

There were twenty-one cases of chronic bilious diarrhoea in Europeans, some of whom were old residents, others new arrivals. This diarrhoea was difficult to account for unless on the supposition that it was a form of sprue. It was certainly not due to *Entamoeba histolytica*, as in no instances was this organism found in the stools, nor was the course of the illness influenced, as far as could be ascertained, by emetine injections. Many of the symptoms of sprue were present, such as the large frothy stools, the early morning diarrhoea, flatulence, dyspepsia, sense of relief and exhaustion following the passage of the stools and rapid emaciation. On the other hand, there were no sprue-like tongue symptoms and, save in one case, no aphthae. The tongue at first was rough and irritated probably owing to some reflex change. The massive stools were of porridgy consistency, resembling nothing so much as a " cowpat." European planters mostly below thirty years of age formed the great majority—sixteen—of the cases: the remaining five occurred in young European ladies, in one of whom diarrhoea commenced after only six weeks residence in Ceylon.

Some of these patients became really acutely ill. They mostly complained of severe dyspepsia accompanied by flatulence partially relieved by passage of stool. There was a variable degree of anaemia of the chlorotic type. In several the haemoglobin percentage was about 70. There were few physical signs. The liver was if anything enlarged but not tender; the abdomen, owing to gaseous dilatation of the intestines and stomach, was swollen and tympanitic. Beyond these indefinite signs nothing further of importance could be made out.

I was unable to ascertain any connection between these cases, which were found scattered all over the country, and the nature of the water supply, or the housing conditions; only eight of the twenty-one lived in houses in which " dry-rot " was evident.

I had no definite means of ascertaining whether these are cases of what is termed in India hill diarrhoea, or whether they are simply early cases of sprue. It is true that in fourteen instances the illness was contracted at and above 4000 ft.[1] but in the remaining seven it

---

[1] Out of twenty-one cases of chronic diarrhoea

3 contracted the disease in the low-country.			
2	,,	,,	between 1000–2000 ft.
1	,,	,,	,, 2000–3000 ft.
2	,,	,,	,, 3000–4000 ft.
10	,,	,,	,, 4000–5000 ft.
3	,,	,,	,, 5000–6000 ft.

developed at a lower elevation. If these were really cases of " hill
diarrhoea," how comes it that the numerous visitors who flock in
hundreds to that popular hill station, Nuwara Eliya (6200 ft.), are not
attacked in the same way? Diarrhoea cases of this description are
certainly rare in that health resort, and after extensive enquiries I
concluded that anything resembling the epidemics of the Indian hill
stations was quite unknown in Ceylon. As additional evidence of the
identity of this diarrhoea and sprue I found that marked improvement
ensued immediately rest in bed and an appropriate milk diet were
enforced and that, except in one instance, removal to sea level was
quite unnecessary to complete the cure. I found that in many cases
of undoubted sprue the illness began with an attack of bilious diarrhoea
of this nature. I think, therefore, that there is every reason for regarding this chronic bilious diarrhoea as being aetiologically identical with
the more typical kind of sprue.

Subgroup 3. *Tongue sprue*

In order to ascertain the frequency of sprue amongst the Ceylon
natives and other races, and in order to be able to interpret the many
tongue conditions found amongst them, I made a careful examination
of a large number of tongues. I shall classify the changes observed
as follows:

1. Conditions associated with hypertrophy of the papillae.
2. Conditions associated with atrophy of the papillae.

1. *Conditions associated with hypertrophy of the papillae*

Under this I include the condition I have termed *the irritated
tongue*. This is a rugged tongue in which, although the changes
in the papillae may be in part of reflex origin, there is generally
some superadded local irritation, such as decayed teeth, pyorrhoea
or other evidences of oral sepsis in combination with some digestive
disturbance. In this condition all the papillae, but more especially
the fungiform, appear prominent and elongated, and have been appropriately termed " stags horn papillae." Tongues of this kind are
commonly met with in Ceylon tea planters inhabiting " dry-rot "
bungalows.

An irritated tongue is seen in many natives addicted to the chewing
of betel—a bolus made up of several irritating ingredients, notably
lime, the leaf of a pepper plant (*Piper betel*) and a fragment of the fruit

of the areca palm (*Areca catechu*). As a result of this habit the tongue, teeth and expectoration are stained a brick-red colour. The frequency of epithelioma of the gums and cheek in those addicted to this practice may be attributable in part to its irritating effects.

The smoker's tongue. Two European gentlemen were met with in whom the constant smoking of strong pipe-tobacco had induced an irritated condition of the tongue. The fungiform papillae were red and inflamed and there was a patch of leucoplakia where the tobacco smoke impinged on the tongue. In both cases the condition caused considerable inconvenience, especially when curries or some other hot substance were partaken of. The pathological changes in the tongue could not be ascribed to any of the ordinary septic processes, as one of these gentlemen had had all his teeth removed several years before, and the other had perfectly sound teeth and healthy gums.

The abnormal tongue. There is yet another condition of the tongue which is commonly met with in native races, especially in the Sinhalese, and is apparently a normal condition. In this the fungiform papillae are hypertrophied and prominent, but are neither red nor inflamed; the filiform papillae, on the other hand, are not in any way affected (Plate I, fig. 13).

2. *Conditions associated with atrophy of the papillae*

The geographical tongue. This was seen in two children. In these instances the process appeared to consist in a desquamation at the tip of the tongue of the surface layers of the fungiform and filiform papillae. Spreading laterally it produced the curious appearance which has been somewhat fancifully compared to a map. In one patient the condition seemed to occasion some slight inconvenience, but in the other no symptoms were noted. Apparently it had no pathological importance.

The syphilitic tongue. Syphilis is a common disease of the Sinhalese, but more especially of the Tamil estate coolie. Secondary and tertiary tongue lesions are common enough amongst them. The general appearance of the syphilitic tongue is so well known as to require no description here, suffice it to say that in the tertiary phase it is red and inflamed, the surface glazed, with leucoplakia in patches, devoid of papillae, the whole organ distorted and deformed by deep fissures and perhaps ulcerated. Of course other syphilitic stigmata may be present elsewhere.

Atrophy of the lingual papillae in chronic wasting disease. In the terminal stages of many wasting diseases, such as phthisis and even in bronchitis and emphysema (one case) in natives, I observed smooth and glazed tongues covered with vestiges of papillae and associated with white crescent-shaped patches of thrush fungus. They were noted most commonly in cachetic native children in the Children's Hospital in Colombo. The little patients, as a rule, suffered from uncontrollable diarrhoea and their mouths and tongues were overgrown with thrush fungus.

Atrophy of the lingual papillae in the anaemias

Ankylostomiasis. I examined a great number of natives suffering from ankylostomiasis, the diagnosis being confirmed by microscopical examination of the stools.

Many of these were very emaciated and suffered intermittently from diarrhoea. In consequence of the anaemia the tongue presented a very pale and flabby appearance. In some instances the filiform papillae were completely atrophied (Plate I, fig. 2), while the fungiform remained as prominent points on a glazed and sometimes superficially fissured surface. I experienced considerable difficulty in ascertaining whether this condition gave rise to any inconvenience. I was able to interview several educated Sinhalese affected in this way who stated that they were unable on account of the soreness of the tongue to continue their favourite habit of betel chewing. I think that when the destruction of the lingual papillae has proceeded to a certain degree and the nerve endings have been exposed, considerable inconvenience is experienced by the patient. In acute ankylostomiasis accompanied by oedema and heart failure atrophy of the lingual papillae was not observed.

Pernicious anaemia. An atrophy of the lingual papillae occurs in other kinds of anaemic disease. Hunter observed occasionally in the terminal stages of pernicious anaemia a raw and fissured tongue and a soreness of the gums. I have recently seen a fatal case of this disease, in which the papillae at the tip of the tongue could be distinguished only with difficulty. Hunter asserts that in microscopical sections a considerable denudation of the surface epithelium can be made out. This feature was not so well marked in the sections of pernicious anaemia tongues which I have had the opportunity of myself examining.

Chlorosis. I saw a young lady who had suffered from chlorosis for a number of years before coming to Ceylon. On the dorsal surface of her tongue there were several patches devoid of papillae, so sensitive as to prevent her from partaking of any acid fruit or spicy substances. I inferred that the atrophy of the papillae in this instance is of the same nature as in pernicious anaemia.

Malaria. A superficially fissured and denuded tongue almost identical with that of chronic ankylostomiasis is often seen in the subjects of a chronic malaria infection.

The leucomatous tongue. I frequently encountered amongst the natives, and especially amongst prisoners and hospital patients, a tongue covered with a peculiar white and filmy deposit, which resembled the drawings of the " leucomatous tongue " in Butlin and Spencer's monograph. It was associated frequently with subacute stomatitis and inflammation of the whole buccal mucous membrane, and a fissured and often raw condition of the angles of the mouth (Plate I, fig. 17).

Sprue

The sprue tongue. For the purpose of description I shall classify my observations under two headings according to the stages of the disease in which the characteristic changes occurred.

Acute stage. The sides or the tip of the tongue are the parts first attacked. The initial lesion is generally of the nature of a diffuse inflammation especially involving the fungiform papillae, which become swollen and prominent. When viewed with a lens the dilated central capillary vessels of the papillae can be clearly seen beneath the smooth and highly polished epithelial coat. At this stage yellow aphthous ulcers, about the size of a millet seed, may appear in the centre of the affected area (Plate I, fig. 3). In two cases I was able to observe the continued effect on the lingual papillae of this inflammatory change over a period of several months. I found that after the subsidence of the inflammation a bare area, quite devoid of papillae, remained to mark its former site (Plate I, fig. 4). After several such inflammatory attacks all the filiform papillae at the sides of the tongue were destroyed and the fungiform, especially those on the anterior portion, became prominent red spots (Plate I, fig. 8). In two instances dark red herpetic vesicles, apparently caused by haemorrhage into the corium of a fungiform papilla, were noted, an occurrence to which Carnegie-Brown has also drawn attention (Plate I, fig. 6).

Chronic stage. After recurring attacks of this specific inflammation all the filiform papillae on the dorsal surface of the tongue are destroyed, the swollen and injected fungiform papillae alone remaining (Plate I, fig. 7). In time the latter are also destroyed and ultimately are represented only by their highly polished pedicles. At this stage longitudinal and often transverse superficial fissures appear and may actually cause the curious chequer-board appearance so often seen in chronic cases. The buccal mucous membrane also presents a highly polished appearance and apparently participates in the chronic inflammation; the lymphoid tissue is also involved causing granular appearances of the hard palate and a shotty condition of the follicles on the inner surface of the lower lip.

In the fatal cases no deep ulceration of the palate or of the undersurface of the tongue was ever seen. The mucous membrane at the angles of the mouth may be similarly affected, sometimes even cracks and fissures appear in this situation causing the patient considerable inconvenience; this is especially noticeable in cases dying of the disease, the interior of whose mouths was covered with the thrush fungus (Plate I, fig. 9). I need hardly point out that the degree of anaemia present greatly affects the general appearance of the tongue; if the anaemia is pronounced the tongue may resemble a piece of yellow cartilage and presents an appearance totally different from that of a non-anaemic case, though the degree of specific change may be the same in both (Plate I, fig. 10). I wish to lay special stress on this point. The effects and extent of the specific sprue inflammation of the tongue vary widely. For instance the tongue changes may not be evident till late in the course of the disease. They may be slight or very severe, transient or persistent, early or late in their occurrence, superficial or more profound. I was able to watch one case in which a fatal termination occurred *one and a half years subsequent to the first onset of symptoms*, and in which no destruction of the lingual papillae took place until during the last few months of life.

It has been suggested by some, notably by Goadby, that the sprue inflammation of the tongue is always associated with pyorrhoea alveolaris; I therefore examined the condition of the gums and their relation to the tongue symptoms in forty-five cases with the following result: the gums and teeth were perfectly healthy in twenty-one; in eleven all teeth had been removed and a false set substituted; in eight only was there an associated pyorrhoea alveolaris; in four the teeth were carious. These figures certainly indicate no intimate association between the condition of the tongue and that of the teeth or gums.

The sprue tongue is so essentially a clean tongue that I rarely observed any " fur " such as would indicate an accumulation of epithelial débris or of bacterial growth on its surface save on the posterior portion where no destruction of the papillae had taken place. This furring is apt to occur during periods of temporary constipation.

Regeneration of the lingual papillae. In examining the tongues of past subjects of sprue and in whom for many years there had been no recurrence of symptoms, I was struck by the normal appearance of the tongue. In the majority of cases it was completely clothed with papillae, while in others there were patches in which the papillae were absent and there may have been slight fissures (Plate I, fig. 5). I was able to observe the process of regeneration of the papillae in one case. This patient had suffered from tongue symptoms for several years; the organ was glazed and the remains of the fungiform papillae alone were distinguishable. After a three months treatment in hospital and a general improvement the filiform papillae had to a large extent reappeared (Plate I, figs. 12 and 14). Unfortunately I was unable to keep the patient any longer under observation, and cannot say if the regeneration was quite complete or permanent.

Aphthae. In association with the sprue tongue small painful aphthous ulcers were commonly observed in the mouth. Their exact situation varied; most commonly they occurred near the opening of Stenson's duct opposite the second upper molar tooth. Sometimes they were found on the inner margin of the lower lip, on the palate, often at the tip of the tongue (Plate I, fig. 11), but only once on the under surface. They varied considerably in size from small yellow points the size of a millet seed to rather irregular ulcers nearly as large as a three-penny piece with a superficial yellow basal slough. As already related, these aphthous ulcers were not found in every case of sprue, even with marked tongue symptoms. Some investigators are inclined to regard these buccal aphthae as the essential lesion of sprue, and consequently entertain expectations of finding in them the specific germ of the disease. I cannot, however, concur in this. I am at a loss as to the exact significance of these lesions in patients long after apparent recovery from sprue. I can cite two such cases. One, a gentleman from the Malay States, who had suffered from sprue in 1908 and who on a milk and fruit diet made a good recovery in England. He had had no sprue symptoms for at least two years when he consulted me, nevertheless aphthous ulcers, frequently of a large size, constantly recurred on the mucous membrane of the cheek and on the inside of the lower lip. The other patient, a lady, had been free from symptoms for a similar period after a cure in Europe, but when I saw her she had an ulcer, about the size of a pea, on the buccal mucous membrane and opposite the second upper molar tooth.

Buccal ulcers apparently identical with sprue aphthae, but to which no diagnostic significance could be attached, were seen in normal Europeans otherwise in perfect health. They were specially persistent in some cases. For instance one gentleman, who consulted me on account of these aphthae, informed me that for the previous four years these lesions had constantly recurred on the buccal mucous membrane and lower lip; his tongue and buccal mucosa were otherwise perfectly normal. I also saw a Sinhalese otherwise in good health with exactly similar and painful lesions. In both cases the aphthae were rapidly cured by the application of the silver nitrate stick.

Tongue sprue in Europeans. As a rule the condition of the tongue just described is associated with symptoms of gastric and intestinal trouble. But this association is by no means invariable. I have met with a considerable number of cases in Ceylon of Europeans, males and females, in whom the only manifestation of sprue was the tongue— "Tongue Sprue" (Plate I, fig. 16). It was not associated with syphilis, tobacco or any local inflammatory condition of the teeth, gums or throat. Of the cases recorded by me below the symptoms commenced in the low-country in two, in the remainder at varying altitudes above 1000 ft.

(1) A middle-aged planter consulted me on account of a painful condition of his tongue of over five months' duration and which prevented him from smoking and from eating highly flavoured articles of food. There was no history of buccal ulceration. The tongue was superficially fissured; the filiform papillae atrophied, the fungiform prominent. There was no question of specific disease, no anaemia or any history of diarrhoea or of other digestive disturbance. Teeth were good and no local irritative focus could be found in the mouth; I watched this patient for over a year and he remained in excellent health, though the tongue changes appeared to be progressive.

(2) A single lady, aged 73, had complained of a sore tongue for over ten years, and was unable, on account of it, to eat curries or acid fruits. There was no history of buccal ulceration. All the teeth had been removed and the sockets were perfectly healthy. So characteristic was the appearance of the tongue that her case had been diagnosed as sprue on several occasions. The tongue was superficially fissured and there was complete absence of the filiform and a corresponding prominence of the fungiform papillae. There was a history of occasional attacks of diarrhoea, but no emaciation or anaemia.

(3) A young planter contracted a sore tongue while resident in the Northern Province. There were periodical remissions and exacerbations of the glossitis, which especially affected the lateral borders where considerable destruction of the filiform papillae had taken place. After being treated for an attack of malaria

and living for some time on a milk diet, the soreness of his tongue abated. There was no history of diarrhoea or other digestive disturbance.

(4) I saw another elderly married lady, long resident in Ceylon, who for seven years had had a condition of the tongue similar to that described in case (2), and which prevented her from partaking of curry or fruit. Salivation was excessive and there was a history of continued buccal ulceration. Her teeth had all been removed. Again in this instance there was no anaemia or digestive disturbance.

(5) Another married lady consulted me for a somewhat similar condition of five years' duration, which prevented her from partaking of highly salted or spiced articles of food. There was no history of diarrhoea, and there was certainly no anaemia. The tongue was slightly fissured; the filiform papillae were partially atrophied, the fungiform inflamed and prominent.

(6) This case occurred in another married lady who had lived all her life in Ceylon. Some six years before I saw her, her tongue became sore and caused her considerable discomfort. Her teeth had all been removed previously. There was no digestive disturbance of any sort. Three years before I saw her, her illness had been diagnosed as sprue, and she had been dieted ever since with the result that the condition rapidly improved and the tongue presented a perfectly normal appearance when I saw her.

(7) A married lady, only two years resident in Ceylon, had an attack of dysentery shortly after her arrival. Since that time she had suffered from occasional diarrhoea attacks. Her teeth had all been removed. Two months before she consulted me her tongue had become inflamed and very tender. No history of aphthae could be obtained. The tongue presented the same appearance as in other cases, that is to say—superficial fissuring, atrophy of the filiform and prominence of the fungiform papillae. On taking a trip to Europe the condition much improved.

Further evidence for regarding this tongue condition as a local manifestation of sprue

I obtained histories of several other Europeans afflicted with a tongue of this description, which may be regarded as throwing further light on its association with sprue proper, and which, moreover, may be quoted with some justification as evidence of the infective nature of the disease.

(A) Husband and wife both afflicted with sore tongues. The wife had suffered much inconvenience from the state of her tongue ever since marriage two years previously; the husband's glossitis antedated that of the wife's by five months.

(B) A single lady, aged sixty-nine, had suffered from a sore tongue for seven years. Her daughter-in-law, who lived in the same house, was affected in a similar way. The former suffered frequently from aphthae on her tongue and cheeks, and for this reason had had all her teeth removed.

(C) An elderly single lady developed a sore tongue and mouth whilst living in the same bungalow with a planter who subsequently contracted sprue and had to leave the Colony on that account.

(D) A married lady developed a sore tongue in August 1912, and at the same time one of the superintendents of the estate, and living in the same bungalow, contracted typical sprue for which he was subsequently treated in England.

Tongue sprue in Burghers. My interest in these tongues was further aroused by the discovery of a similar condition in three generations of a family of high-class Colombo and Kandy Burghers. I met with the disease in three ladies of this family, two sisters and a niece. Syphilis, carious teeth and pyorrhoea alveolaris could be excluded. None of them complained of any digestive or other symptoms. Their family history, which they gave me in full detail, showed that members had for several generations suffered acutely from or had died of some form of diarrhoea, probably sprue, while others had suffered solely from sore tongue.

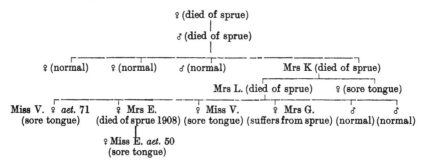

Though it is possible that the details of the previous generations are unreliable, the facts, in so far as they concern the present one, may be regarded as correct and as affording a presumption that the association of typical sprue with the sore tongues in associated members of the same family is more than a coincidence.

Tongue sprue in natives. A similar condition of the tongue is extremely prevalent amongst prisoners and is familiar to the prison officials in Ceylon. Prisoners so affected are recognised by their inability to partake of their curry stuffs, of which they are inordinately fond. The appearance of these tongues varies widely according to the stage the disease process has reached. In the most advanced cases the stripping of the epithelium is quite complete and leaves a raw glazed and superficially fissured tongue, such as is illustrated in the plate (Plate I, fig. 15). This is often combined with a polished buccal mucous membrane and a cracked and leucoplakic condition of the angles of the mouth. The teeth and gums may be and usually are perfectly normal. From a number of observations I made on these tongues the process appeared to have begun at the tip and to have spread backwards.

The disease is common to both sexes and to the several races— Sinhalese, Tamils, Javanese and Malays—found in Ceylon. It would serve no useful purpose to detail in this place all the observations on which these statements are based; I have included these in the Appendix (see Appendix VII). Suffice it to say that I found these tongues in 16 per cent. of ordinary non-criminal Tamil coolie estate labourers, also in a number of hospital patients, but by far the most commonly in prisoners and in every part of Ceylon visited (14·7 per cent. in Colombo and 22 per cent. in Anuradhapura gaol).

According to the evidence of prison medical officers the disease appears to be of an infectious nature and when once introduced to spread with great rapidity. It is commoner in long sentence prisoners than in new arrivals (Plate I, fig. 15).

In none of the cases, or only very exceptionally, was a history of diarrhoea obtainable and there was no anaemia. The haemoglobin percentage, which was estimated whenever possible, averaged about 80.

It may be urged by some that this is but a symptom of scurvy, as it is supposed to be associated with the consumption of dried fish, a staple and favourite Sinhalese article of diet, but other symptoms of that disease, such as haemorrhages and spungy gums, were absent. Neither is there any valid reason for regarding it as depending on dried fish as some have suggested, seeing that it is prevalent in Jaffna gaol where a diet of fresh fish as being more economical is substituted for the dried article in use elsewhere. In Jaffna the prison diet is a very liberal one, consisting of rice, vegetables, meat, fish and dahl (pulse). Since neither betel nor tobacco is permitted in prison, these habits cannot conduce to or induce the condition. The suggestion may be made that this glossitis may be merely a symptom of pellagra, a disease in which denudation of the tongue epithelium takes place during the terminal stages, especially when associated with a frothy diarrhoea. But against such a supposition I would urge that no symptoms of insanity or the peculiar cutaneous manifestations so characteristic of pellagra were apparent in any of these prisoners.

The possibility of these tongues being merely a tertiary manifestation of syphilis had to be considered. (*Vide* Appendix VIII.) Thirty-one cases were tested by the Noguchi modification of the Wassermann reaction, but only in five instances was a positive result obtained.

When the frequency of syphilis amongst these natives is considered this is not an undue proportion of positive results, and therefore syphilis may be excluded as a cause.

This tongue disease is not confined to the prisons nor to coolie lines. I found an exactly similar tongue in a high caste young Tamil who was attending a high-class school in Jaffna.

As additional evidence of the connection of this bare tongue with that of true sprue, I was fortunate enough to obtain a post-mortem on a woman who exhibited tongue symptoms during life, and who subsequently died from some superadded tubercular infection. The pathological changes I found in sections of her tongue resembled in every respect those in the tongue of true sprue.

An acute and apparently septic stomatitis associated with a purulent infection of the gums and an acute inflammation of the buccal mucous membrane, but unaccompanied by a stripping of the epithelium or a destruction of the papillae, is also found in these natives and appears to be an entirely separate affection.

It is customary in the gaols to employ native remedies for the treatment of these sore tongues. The substitution of half-cooked liver or liver soup for their curry and rice is regarded by the prisoners as a valuable remedy. But a still more effective one in their estimation are the leaves of the " Kathiri-murunga " (*Sebania grandiflora*), a small tree grown in every prison courtyard. These leaves are either chewed raw or are partaken of as a vegetable with rice. The plantation coolies are in the habit of chewing, also as a remedial measure, the leaves of the " Gotagola " (*Hydrocotyle javanica* and *asiatica*), small plants which flourish amongst the tea bushes. As far as I was able to gather, the native doctors or " Vederalas " are in the habit of pre-scribing these same remedies for sprue in natives and they have been adopted also by fully qualified Ceylonese practitioners for the routine treatment of this disease.

The clinical and epidemiological evidence I have recounted suggests the conclusions (a) that sprue is a specific germ-caused disease, (b) that the "sore sprue tongues" of the European and of the native are identical, (c) and that it is an active process ; and (d) it is not the same as the atrophic bare tongue of ankylostomiasis, of malaria and of pernicious anaemia which latter may be regarded as the result of deficient nutrition and as a passive condition.

CHAPTER XIII

INVESTIGATIONS ON THE CLINICAL PATHOLOGY OF SPRUE

Stools. The typical sprue stool has peculiarities, obvious even to the untrained eye, to which a certain amount of aetiological import has been attached.

The three important features of the sprue stool are their colour, their size and their chemical composition. I propose to consider very briefly under these headings the results of numerous observations and analyses. The analytical methods I employed have been taken from Strasburger's monograph *Die Fäzes des Menschen*, 1910, and Harley and Goodbody's *Chemical Investigation of Gastric and Intestinal Diseases*, 1906, to both of which I am indebted for much information.

Colour. It is a matter of common observation that the character of the food has a great influence on the colour of the stools. According to Strasburger, the stools are brown on a mixed diet, a darker brown on a pure meat diet, green on a vegetable diet (the green colour being partly due to chlorophyll and partly to bacterial action), and orange to light yellow on a milk diet. The intensity of colour is further influenced by the length of time the faeces have remained in the intestinal canal. Though these factors play an important part in the coloration of the stools, yet the composition of the bile pigments plays a still more important one; the common pigment of the stools is hydro-bilirubin, or stercobilin (isomeric with urobilin, the urinary pigment and a reduction product of bilirubin), recognisable by its spectrum and certain chemical reactions.

It was formerly stated that the large and frothy stools passed in the early stages of sprue are abnormally rich in bile constituents, but that as the disease progresses these become reduced in amount and eventually are absent altogether. It was generally held that to this peculiarity the white colour of the sprue stool was due. Brunton, on the other hand, ascribed the pale colour mainly to a large percentage of crystalline fat. Later analyses by Sidney Martin showed that the bile constituents, such as the bile acids (glycocholate and taurocholate of soda) were present, and still more recently it was proved by Blyth that the bile pigments were really present but in the form of a colourless compound called leucourobilin[1] (Nencki), a reduction product of hydrobilirubin.

According to Walker[2] such a reduction of the normal bile pigments occurs in certain diseases (*e.g.*, malignant disease of the pancreas) in which the pancreatic juice is either not secreted or is unable to enter the intestinal canal, and Mayo Robson[3] asserts that the faeces of interstitial pancreatitis may resemble both in colour and size those of sprue.

It is therefore now fully recognised that the bile elements in the sprue faeces are either by reason of the liver atrophy much diminished in amount, or that in the presence of some unknown factor (such as the absence of the pancreatic ferments), the pigments have undergone some chemical change resulting in a colourless compound. It is now believed that it is partly to diminished bile secretion (or to chemically altered bile) and partly to the abnormal proportion of crystalline fats that the pale colour of the sprue faeces is to be ascribed.

In a proportion of my cases, particularly in my early cases of sprue which were partaking of a mixed diet, I failed to find the typical white-wash stools described in text-books. Eleven acute cases were seen at a fairly early stage and the colour of their stools noted. In five the colour was light brown; in one greenish-yellow; and in three light-yellow. I have notes of one case in which the stools remained of a brick-red colour throughout the patient's ultimately fatal illness and even when she was living on a pure milk diet. In the more chronic cases I observed the typical *chalky stools* only when milk and farinaceous foods composed the greater part of the patient's dietary.

I was able in two fatal cases to ascertain that the liquid greyish-brown stools, passed involuntarily a few days before death, contained unaltered biliverdin and therefore gave a positive Gmelin's test, a reaction which was also obtained in the stools of a third sprue patient during an acute attack of diarrhoea.

Further observations on these pigments were made in four of my

---

[1] According to Strasburger, leucourobilin is identical with urobilinogen and can be detected by the formation of a red precipitate on the addition of a few drops of zinc chloride to an ammoniacal extract of the faeces. I have obtained this result many times, but it was impossible to exclude the presence of indol or skatol which also give the same reaction.

[2] Walker (1889), *Med. Chir. Trans.* LXIII, p. 257.

[3] Mayo Robson and Cammidge (1907), *The Pancreas, its Surgery and Pathology*.

patients. For a period of two to three months the stools were analysed almost daily. In these sprue stools I found that Schmidt's test for hydrobilirubin became positive, only, if previous to the test the faeces had been exposed for some time to the air, but even then the red colour resulting from the reaction did not become apparent till an hour or more had elapsed after the admixture of the corrosive sublimate solution. The exact time at which the reaction became positive varied within wide limits in different cases and from day to day. I found that, if some of the pasty white stool be cut across, the central portion was white, while the outer layers having become oxidized had assumed a yellow colour. If the faeces of the central white area be treated with 90 per cent. alcohol and filtered, a white colourless fluid results which slowly assumes a deeper shade after contact with the air. Should the test tube containing this filtrate be exposed to sunlight or be shaken up with air, this colour change takes place more rapidly; the same effect is produced by the addition of a drop of nitric acid or of iodine. I was unable to detect in the colourless solution the characteristic spectroscopic bands of hydrobilirubin until it had become a darker colour. I think there is some justification for concluding that hydrobilirubin is present in sprue faeces, but that the greater part is reduced to the colourless form called leucourobilin, and that the oxidation of this substance to hydrobilirubin[1] readily takes place in the faeces on exposure to the air outside the body. That normal bile is secreted in sprue is evident from two post-mortems I performed, in which I found abundant amber-coloured bile in the gall bladder. Any normal chemical change in the composition of the bile pigments must therefore take place during the passage of the faecal matter through the intestinal canal.

By employing Pettenkoffer's test, bile acids were found in seven out of eleven acute sprue stools and were constantly present in the more solid stools of four of my patients undergoing treatment. No traces of blood pigments were ever found.

The results of the chemical reactions of the sprue stools were compared with those I found in other conditions. In nine normal stools a hydrobilirubin reaction was present in all and a bile acid reaction in eight; biliverdin and bilirubin were absent entirely. In four cases of ankylostomiasis, hydrobilirubin was present in two, and a bile acid reaction only in one; while in four cases of amoebic dysentery the hydrobilirubin reaction was positive in three and a bile acid reaction in one.

---

[1] An excellent account of the chemistry of leucourobilin and hydrobilirubin in sprue is given by Van der Scheer in Mense's *Handb. der Tropenk.* 1905, II. 26, and agrees in the main with the conclusions arrived at in this paper. The reader should note that Justi also in a recent post-mortem found bile in the gall bladder and unaltered biliverdin in the diarrhoeic stools of sprue before death.

Size of sprue stools. From observations I made on the stools of
five patients undergoing treatment, I found that not only did the amount
of excrement vary considerably from day to day, but also when the
total amount was estimated over successive long periods. In my
cases the average daily quantity passed varied from 173 grammes
to 411 grammes, according to the severity of the disease process and
the progress of the patient under treatment. The smallest individual
daily stool recorded by me was 56 grammes, the largest 901 grammes.
(In Harley's published sprue case the average daily quantity passed
was 255 grammes, but varied between the extremes of 120 and 337
grammes.)

Details of the amount of stool passed, together with the quantity of food ingested,
will be found in Appendix XV. In the first case therein narrated the disease had
been of considerable duration, but with appropriate treatment great improvement
ensued. The average weight of stool passed, estimated over a period of forty days,
was 411 grammes. In the second case the disease was typical. The patient, over
middle age, improved rapidly under treatment. The stools averaged 352 grammes
over a period of thirty days. In the third case tongue symptoms were entirely
absent. There was considerable improvement under treatment. The average
weight of the entire stool over a period of twenty-two days was 308 grammes.
The fourth case was an old man of seventy in whom the disease had been of considerable duration. An average of 363 grammes of stool was passed over a period
of thirty-seven days. The fifth case was a young and vigorous man in whom
recovery was phenomenally rapid. The average amount of stool passed over a
period of forty-four days was 173 grammes.

In the normal healthy subject the weight of the stool varies with
the nature and amount of food. According to Rubner, on a milk diet
of 3075 grammes total weight, and containing about 307 grammes of
solids, the average total weight of stool is 174 grammes (= 40 grammes
total solids). According to Harley, on a diet of 2291 grammes (containing
229 grammes solids) the total weight of stool is 135·2 grammes, in other
words 87 per cent. the amount of solid matter ingested in the food
is normally absorbed. In sprue I found that the relationship between
the quantity of food ingested and the amount of solids excreted varied
considerably in individual cases. In one case in particular, at an
early stage of treatment, the average amount of food ingested daily
over a period of one week (milk and fruit diet) was 859 grammes total
weight (containing about 160 grammes solids) and the total weight
of stool passed was 259 grammes (= 59·5 grammes solids), or in other
words 64 per cent. of the solids ingested were absorbed at a time when
the patient was rapidly gaining in body weight. In another case of a

much more chronic nature and also on a milk and fruit daily diet of 2271 grammes (containing 422 grammes solids), 303 grammes total weight of stool (= 75·5 grammes solids) were passed, that is to say out of the amount of ingested solids 82 per cent. had been absorbed. The quantity of stool in this case increased in direct proportion to the amount of the diet ingested, for on a diet weighing 3136 grammes (containing 651·1 grammes solids) the average daily weight of the stool increased, when estimated over a period of a week, to 350 grammes total weight (= 87·5 grammes solids).

As may be inferred, an increase in the weight of any patient undergoing treatment bears a direct relation to the amount of stool passed. For instance, in one case the average gain in body weight over a period of one week was 161 grammes per diem, and the average amount of stool passed per diem 605 grammes; during a subsequent week, when a distinct improvement in the patient's condition was manifest, the daily increase in body weight had almost doubled to 377 grammes, and the amount of stool had fallen to 347 grammes, that is to almost half the daily average of the previous week. These figures seem to indicate that the loss of body weight in sprue and the large size of the excreta passed is due to some deficiency in the power of assimilation and that any increase in the patient's body weight can be attributed directly to an improvement in the powers of digestion and absorption.

The average daily stool excretion is naturally dependent on the number of the stools and the amount of contained fluid. The liquid diarrhoeic stools which necessarily contain a large amount are quite unsuitable for analysis, but it was instructive to estimate the proportion of contained fluid in the more solid pasty sprue stools. Four stools were accordingly analysed with apparently similar results in each instance, the amount of solid matter resulting from the dried stools was found to be just one-quarter of the original weight and they therefore contained 75 per cent. of water, a result which compares favourably with 77 per cent. given by Harley for a milk diet stool in the normal subject.

(1) *Chemical composition of the stools*

Amount of fat. The quantity of fat in sprue stools can be roughly gauged by a simple microscopical examination. On a milk diet numerous needles of crystalline fats and soaps invariably can be seen in the stool, and in a smear preparation treated with osmic acid the particles of fat become discernible as dark microscopic globules. The amount of fat in the dried faeces can be more exactly estimated by means of a Soxhlet apparatus; by this means the percentage was found to vary in different specimens from 3·5 per cent. to 24·2 per cent. of the total dried residue.

According to Harley's analysis the amount of fat in the faeces of a normal subject fed on 1½ to 3 pints of milk per diem is about 3·75 grammes. The amount passed in the faeces by four of my sprue patients[1] was greatly in excess of the normal and varied from 6·4 to 30·2 grammes per diem.

These figures indicate that sprue faeces contain considerably more than double the normal amount of fat, results more or less in agreement with similar analyses by Harley and in which, though the amount of fat passed in the stools varied from day to day, the average quantity for three days was found to be 35·92 grammes.

The amount of fat absorbed in my sprue cases could be estimated as varying from 70 to 90 per cent. of the total ingested fat, figures higher than Harley's 53 per cent., but approximating to those given by Van der Scheer.

These investigations all tend to confirm the statement, so generally accepted, that the process of fat digestion and absorption is in some way markedly affected in sprue, since in the normal subject on a milk diet the fat absorption has been found to be over 95 per cent. of the total amount ingested.

Carbohydrates. Qualitatively, when the patient is on carbohydrates, undigested starch can be demonstrated by the microscopic examination of the stool. In sprue stools, resulting from a milk diet to which toast and bread have been added, undigested starch grains are rendered blue and become very apparent on the addition of iodine to the preparation.

Quantitative estimation of the undigested starch residue can only be roughly performed by Strasburger's simple apparatus. In this

---

[1] The figures are as follows:

(1) On a milk diet of 3 pints the dried stool weighed 183 grammes and contained 6·4 grammes of fat.

(2) On a milk diet of 3½ pints the dried stool weighed 58·8 grammes and contained 10·1 grammes of fat.

(3) On a mixed diet and 3 pints of milk the dried stool weighed 203 grammes and contained 22·2 grammes of fat.

(4) On a mixed diet and 1 pint of milk the dried stool weighed 129 grammes and contained 30·2 grammes of fat.

These figures agree in the main with Van der Scheer's analysis ((1905) *Tijdschr. v. Geneesk.* x. 637, and in Mense's *Handb. der Tropenk.* (1905), ii.).

method a gramme of faeces is mixed with water and placed in a glass bulb to which two gas collecting tubes are affixed. Under normal conditions and after twenty-four hours incubation at 37° C., the limb of the collecting tube ought to be half full of gas, but from a sprue stool almost double the normal quantity of gas was produced. The method gives but a very rough estimation, as a given quantity of starch is fermented to a different degree by different species of bacteria and consequently with varying gas production.

Reaction of sprue stools. According to Strasburger the nature of the diet has an influence on the resulting reaction of the normal stool which is alkaline on a milk and meat diet and neutral on a mixed diet. Apparently a deficiency of acid gastric secretion has no influence on the consequent reaction of the faeces.

It is an accepted fact that, irrespective of the nature of the diet, the typical sprue stools are almost invariably acid to litmus paper; in Ceylon I found the reaction invariably acid in eleven acute cases, alkaline only in two. The reaction of the stools of patients undergoing treatment varies slightly from day to day. In one case it became alkaline after the patient's first fortnight in hospital and when he was on the highroad to a good recovery; but in the remaining four cases it was almost invariably acid during the whole time I had an opportunity of testing the stools.

Acid stools are not a peculiarity of sprue, for this reaction was obtained in those of chronic diarrhoea, amoebic dysentery and ankylostomiasis. I further found that the acidity of sprue stools is not in any way due to free hydrochloric (di-amido-azo-benzol test), but apparently to the presence of lactic and butyric acids.

The odour of the sprue stools. The odour of the faeces is dependent mainly on the nature of the dietary and of the degree of putrefaction occurring in the large intestine. The sprue stools bear an indefinite, but peculiarly sour odour, graphically described to me by one of my patients as resembling that of burned paint, and possibly due to the chemical changes in the intestinal canal and gases generated by the growth of gas-forming micro-organisms, such as the yeast fungus.

Ferments.

Traces of various intestinal ferments have been found in normal stools, and their presence can be verified by certain fermentation tests. I will first give a summary of our present knowledge of the subject.

According to Strasburger *pepsin* is seldom found in stools of normal consistency, but occurs in those of diarrhoea.

According to Hemmiter and Strasburger traces of *trypsin* are found, but only inconstantly, in normal stools, but after experimental occlusion of the pancreatic duct in dogs it was found to be invariably absent and is therefore probably derived from that secretion.

According to Strasburger the *diastase* or *amylase* in the stools is not derived from the saliva, as when given by the mouth the action of the salivary ferment is neutralised in the intestinal canal; at present it is still a matter of dispute whence it is derived, though experimental work on dogs, as well as observations of diseased conditions of the human pancreas, points to its derivation from the pancreatic juice, and Strasburger, by employing a very delicate technique, has found that it is rarely absent in normal stools.

Von Jaksch found *invertin* in the stools of children. So far there have been no similar investigations on adult stools, but it is inferred that it is derived from the intestinal mucosa and is normally present in adult stools.

By applying the appropriate tests[1], of which I give details below, on seventeen occasions stools from six sprue patients were tested for the presence of these ferments. Traces of *pepsin* were found inconstantly in the stools of all six, but *trypsin* was invariably absent, though I found it in normal stools tested as controls. *Diastase* was found to be constantly present in every sprue stool examined. A saccharose-inverting ferment, presumably *invertin*, was only found in three cases.

The results of this line of investigation, though somewhat indefinite, agree with a similar investigation undertaken by Rademaker, and indicate a diminution in the amount or entire absence of the pancreatic ferments in sprue.

The filtrate of sprue stools were tested for albuminous matter and its derivatives—albumoses and peptones—but with a negative result. The entire absence in the stools of serous matter liable to be derived

---

[1] *Tests for intestinal ferments in the faeces* (Strasburger). An emulsion of the stool in water is made to the consistency of thick cream and is then filtered through fine muslin.

(1) *For Invertin.* A small piece of saccharose and a crystal of thymol is added to filtrate.

(2) *For Diastase.* Starch solution and a crystal of thymol are added to another portion of the filtrate in a similar manner.

(3) *For Trypsin.* A cube of the white of a hard boiled egg, a grain of sodium bicarbonate and a crystal of thymol are added to another portion of the filtrate.

(4) *For Pepsin.* The emulsion of the stool is made with 1 per cent. hydrochloric acid in the place of water and after filtration a cube of hard boiled egg and a crystal of thymol are added.

The test-tubes containing these ingredients are incubated for twenty-four hours at 37° C. and the contents filtered. If *invertin* be present in the first test-tube, reduction of Fehling's solution will take place; if *diastase* be present in the second, the dextrin produced will give a brown reaction with iodine. The third and fourth test-tubes will, if albumoses and peptones be produced, give the biuret reaction.

from any intestinal ulceration is of interest, as probably indicating that intestinal lesions of this nature do not play an essential part in the pathogenesis of this disease.

Mucus in sprue stools. Round the large pasty and rather constipated motions passed during convalescence a coating of thick mucus was occasionally observed; it was never bile stained. Little could be seen by a microscopical examination[1] save vacuolated remains of the intestinal epithelium. No red cells or other evidences of intestinal ulceration were ever observed. In the typical frothy evacuations I failed to find any mucus; therefore I regard the excessive mucus in some cases as of no special significance and as being probably derived from the lower part of the rectum.

(2) *Urine*

Amount. There is little to be said about the total amount of urine passed. In three patients, as a result of daily observations over a period of six weeks, the quantity was found to be about 1600 c.c. per diem, or about the normal amount; in two others, both suffering from intermittent attacks of diarrhoea and who passed a considerable amount of fluid by the bowel, the amount of urine was diminished to an average of 594 and 755 c.c. per diem respectively.

Reaction. This was invariably acid in every case and on every occasion on which it was tested.

Specific gravity. The specific gravity was found to be normal in every instance (1015–1020).

Urea. The daily urea excretion was estimated by Dupré's apparatus. It was found, even when the diet ingested contained the physiological amount of proteids, to be somewhat lower than in the normal subject, and to vary slightly in different cases from a daily average of 20·5 to 25·5 grammes.

The somewhat rough estimations on the proteid content of the ingested milk that I was able to make indicate that the urea in sprue is of exogenous and not of endogenous origin, that is to say, not derived from any excess of tissue metabolism (*vide* Appendix IX). The amount of urea excreted was subject to slight daily variations. In one patient it showed sudden and somewhat unexpected rises during convalescence

---

[1] One gentleman suffering from an attack of subacute sprue passed for a few days in his stools blood and mucus containing amoebae. Under emetine treatment a rapid amelioration took place. I regarded this complication as being due to a superimposed amoebic infection.

and on occasions entailing some extra physical exertion; I attached no special importance to this point.

Inorganic sulphates were found to be invariably present in the normal amount.

Uric acid was also present in the majority of cases.

Indican[1]. An indicanuria in sprue has already been advanced by Rademaker as a diagnostic point. It is of no great significance, seeing that the presence in the urine of these organic sulphates is dependent upon the amount of intestinal putrefaction. I could not, however, obtain an indican reaction in every one of my cases. Only five urines of patients in whom the diarrhoea was acute gave a feeble reaction, but it was most marked in two specimens passed shortly before death. Even when present it is of the most evanescent character; in a period of from two to six days it disappeared entirely from the urine of two of my patients, directly the appropriate treatment had been applied, and, presumably, directly the amount of intestinal putrefaction had been thereby diminished.

Urobilin. This pigment was present in the urines of thirteen anaemic cases and was recognised by its spectrum as well as by fluorescence with zinc chloride in an ammoniacal solution. It also appears to be evanescent and disappeared entirely after the first week in bed and directly the blood condition (as ascertained by numerous blood counts) had begun to improve. It was not found in the urines of all other cases of chronic diarrhoea in which there was no marked degree of anaemia. Its presence in the sprue urine appears to be intimately dependent on the degree of blood destruction in any particular case.

Albumen. Traces of albumen (Heller's ring test) were found in the urine four times, three of which were in women. No other evidence of kidney disease could be obtained and I am inclined to believe that it was of purely fortuitous occurrence.

No traces of sugar or bile were found and the diazo[2] reaction was invariably negative. The urines were generally devoid of sediment; on one occasion only was a deposit of oxalate crystals seen. Tests for acetone and diacetic acids were also invariably negative.

Cammidge's reaction. Much stress has been laid in recent years upon the presence of this reaction in the urine of sprue, especially by

---

[1] I found that the urinary indigogens could be demonstrated by Obermayer's method (lead acetate and chloroform) in cases in which the older method (nitric acid and chloroform) failed.

[2] Justi found the diazo reaction positive in his case during the last few days of life.

Cammidge and Begg[1]. The former found a positive pancreatic reaction in 60 per cent. of sprue urines examined, a discovery which has strengthened the belief that the disease may be due to some affection of the pancreas. In order to verify this point I performed this reaction in twenty-seven sprue urines in Ceylon, in some even on several separate occasions, but in every instance I obtained a negative result. In performing this reaction the technique of the more recent and improved method was carefully followed, as detailed by Cammidge himself[2].

(3) *The saliva of sprue*

Special attention was given to the examination and chemistry of the sprue saliva, a point which has previously been investigated by Van der Scheer, who found the reaction of saliva alkaline to litmus paper in early cases, but acid in the more advanced cases.

In every sprue case I examined, and especially those in whom the tongue symptoms predominated, the saliva presented a marked acid reaction to litmus paper, this was especially noticeable in the advanced cases in whose mouths a deposit of thrush (*Monilia*) was noted. (By inoculating the thrush fungus into alkaline saliva I found a considerable degree of acidity produced by a twenty-four hours' growth.)

The reaction of the inflamed tongue in all cases of tongue sprue was also markedly acid. The prominent fungiform papillae especially gave a marked reaction, so that a piece of blue litmus paper when applied to such a tongue presented a number of red spots, each spot corresponding to an inflamed papilla.

Van Haeften and others have commented on the absence of the potassium sulphocyanide reaction in the sprue saliva. Mense, who made some investigations on this point, found that the amount of this substance even in the saliva of normal individuals varied enormously. In the majority of my sprue cases I found a positive reaction present, and in those cases which I tested with starch a positive ptyalin reaction was also obtained.

(4) *The gastric juice*

The chemistry of the gastric juice in sprue has been investigated by Van der Scheer[3] who found in the majority of cases an increase of free hydrochloric acid, in others a normal amount, while in a few it was entirely absent.

---

[1] Begg (1912), *Sprue, its Diagnosis and Treatment*, 49.

[2] Mayo Robson (1907), *The Pancreas, its Surgery and Pathology*, 252.

[3] Van der Scheer (1905), Mense's *Handb. der Tropenk.* 99.

I had only one opportunity of making such an analysis, free hydro-chloric acid was present and the total acidity amounted to ·4 per cent.

(5)　The blood in sprue

In discussing the anaemia so characteristic of sprue one must necessarily enter into the difficult and much contested question of the intestinal toxaemias. The generation of some bacterial toxin in the intestinal canal and its absorption into the blood stream, is generally urged by modern writers as the most probable cause of such familiar anaemias as chlorosis, pernicious anaemia and the anaemia which accompanies a chronic intestinal stasis. The marked anaemia associated with verminous diseases, such as ankylostome and bothrio-cephalus infections, is now held to be produced by the poisons excreted by these parasites into and absorbed from the intestinal canal, the resulting anaemia being severe in proportion to the amount of toxin produced by the parasites, the length of time the infection has persisted, and individual susceptibility.

We may regard the anaemia of sprue in a similar light, for according to the investigations of Thin, Richartz, Van der Scheer and Low, a grave degree of anaemia is found only in the most advanced stages of the disease. In the early stages there is no alteration either in the number of red or white cells or in their relative proportions, but as the disease progresses the former become profoundly altered both in shape and size and nucleated red cells may even appear; in short the terminal blood picture may resemble that of pernicious anaemia. The lowest blood counts so far recorded in sprue are one by Richartz of 960,000 red cells and 20 per cent. haemoglobin and a second by Low[1] of 1,200,000 red cells and 30 per cent. haemoglobin.

In Appendix X, I have given a number of blood counts of my sprue cases together with a record of the duration of symptoms in each case. The lowest blood counts there recorded are taken from patients just a few weeks before death. Even in these the red cells were never reduced below 1,000,000 per c.mm. or the haemoglobin below 30 per cent.

In some of the native cases, also proving fatal, a low blood cell count and a low haemoglobin percentage were encountered, but in these a co-existing ankylostome infection could not be excluded as a factor in the production of the anaemia.

[1] Low (1912), *Journ. Trop. Med.* 129.

In all these very anaemic cases other evidences of blood degeneration —such as polychromatophilic granules, alteration in size and shape of the red cells—were encountered, but only twice, namely, in a blood smear made from the heart post-mortem and once during the last few days of life, were nucleated red cells met with in any numbers. In fact the blood picture in these two cases save for the absence of megaloblasts resembled that of an advanced pernicious anaemia.

Another fact emerges from the figures I have given, namely, that when pronounced the anaemia is of the pernicious type and the colour index higher than normal. There are, however, some instances where the red cells were normal in number and the haemoglobin considerably reduced. But, though present as a general rule, a great degree of anaemia need not necessarily precede the fatal termination. In Justi's case the red cells numbered 4,600,000 and the haemoglobin 73 per cent. before death; even in one of my fatal cases the red cells never fell below 3,900,000 and at the autopsy an 80 per cent. haemoglobin was found. A total white and differential leucocytic count was made whenever possible, but as these counts do not show any remarkable features, I do not propose to discuss them.

In addition to blood counts, smears were carefully searched for parasites, but always with a negative result. Blood cultures of 2 c.c. of blood drawn from the median bacilic vein and inoculated into agar and broth were made in one case but proved to be sterile; neither was I able to demonstrate in the blood serum any agglutinin specific to any of the numerous bacilli and yeast organisms which I isolated from the saliva and stools.

There is little evidence then for regarding the anaemia of sprue as being otherwise than of secondary origin, due probably to the absorption from the intestinal canal of some blood-destroying toxin.

That a severe degree of anaemia need not necessarily precede the fatal termination is an important point as showing that the anaemia itself is not an essential factor in the disease. It is probable that the exact degree is dependent, as in other well-known anaemias, on certain factors, such as the duration and severity of the intestinal symptoms, the amount of toxin absorbed and the individual susceptibility of the patient.

CHAPTER XIV

THE MORBID ANATOMY AND PATHOLOGY OF SPRUE

(1) *Previous work on the morbid anatomy*

In discussing this difficult question I propose to confine myself to the more recent published descriptions. Although many autopsies were made and described by the old Indian and French authors, yet in the face of the difficulty they encountered in differentiating sprue from dysenteric conditions, and in the absence of any accurate descriptions of the clinical symptoms during the patients' lifetime, we may disregard their evidence for our present purpose.

The confusion which undoubtedly exists with regard to the morbid anatomy of sprue may be explained, in part at any rate, by the fact that so few autopsies have been described and still fewer examined microscopically by more modern methods.

The views of different authors on this subject may be stated briefly as follows. Van der Burg considered the essential lesion to be a gastric catarrh with secondary atrophy of the intestinal walls and of the liver. Manson considered that the disease process especially affected the small intestine which was attenuated to such a great extent as to be diaphanous, the muscular coats to be atrophied and the submucosa infiltrated with round cells. Le Dantec and Scheube also state that the gut wall is thinned and the glandular elements atrophied.

Spencer, Williams and Bassett-Smith, on the other hand, aver that the principal lesion is a fibrosis of the pancreas. This view receives some degree of support from the clinical resemblance of sprue to certain cases of chronic pancreatitis and by the fact that in Cammidge's hands the urine of a proportion of cases gave a positive pancreatic reaction.

The pathological description most often quoted is based on two post-mortem examinations by Thin in the microscopical examination of which he was assisted by Dr Wethered. In the first case there was marked attenuation of the small intestine, but no ulceration; in the second, small erosions were found in the jejunum, together with

ten superficial ulcers in the large intestine. The mucous membrane
was converted into a structureless substance containing leucocytes;
the muscular coats were attenuated. Thin considered that the disease
process was mainly limited to the mucous membrane of the ileum
where it caused destruction of the villi, especially of Lieberkühn's
follicles, and a cystic distension of their lumen. The epithelial lining
of the oesophagus was missing.

In opposition to this are the views of Faber. This investigator
had the opportunity of performing an autopsy in Copenhagen on an
undoubted case of sprue from China, in which many of the tissues
were microscopically examined. The abdominal cavity was injected
with formalin immediately after death and the tissues fixed. Sixteen
ulcerations of Peyer's patches, varying much in size, were found in
the small intestine. An atrophy of the gut wall was not observed.
Microscopically a diffuse inflammation of the mucosa was found throughout the whole length of the gut; frequently round cells were found in
the submucosa as well. The surface epithelium was for the most part
well preserved; there was no cystic dilatation of the Lieberkühn's
follicles. Pancreas, liver and other intestinal glands were normal.

Faber emphasises the difficulty of distinguishing microscopically
between an inflamed and a non-inflamed bowel, as the interstitial
tissue of the villi is normally much infiltrated with round cells, a feature
which in some cases is more pronounced at some times than at others.

Still more recently (December 1913) Justi has published a very
complete account of the macro- and microscopic pathology in one
case, to which frequent allusion will be made later on. His conclusions
are in the main in agreement with those of Faber, that is in regarding
the destruction of the villi and the loss of surface epithelium as a post-
mortem phenomenon, especially liable to occur under tropical conditions.
In this case thinning of the small intestine was found together with
superficial ulceration and thickening of the large intestine; all the
organs were wasted to the same proportional degree.

To arrive at reliable conclusions in the morbid anatomy of sprue it is necessary
to eliminate all factors conducing to post-mortem changes in a structure so delicate
as the intestinal mucosa. In the tropics, in the absence of any refrigerating
apparatus, post-mortem changes make themselves apparent, more especially in the
intestinal tube, with disconcerting rapidity. Many *post-mortem* phenomena such as
loss of surface epithelium have been ascribed to *ante-mortem* changes. In the published
descriptions of the pathology not enough stress has been laid on the importance of
fixing the intestinal mucosa immediately death has taken place. It is also important
to remember that washing out the intestinal tube with water before fixation may

cause considerable distortion and even destruction of the columnar epithelium. Points such as these have been emphasised by Hunter, Faber and Bloch in their studies of the intestinal changes found in pernicious anaemia and in infantile diarrhoea.

In making the autopsies I have described in this paper every precaution has been taken to ward against any such post-mortem changes. The tissues were removed as soon after death as possible (two hours) and immediately fixed in 4 per cent. formalin.

For demonstrating the cytological detail of the alimentary canal I recognise that formalin is an inferior fixative to Zenker's or to Müller's fluids, but in the conditions under which I was working it was found to be the most convenient. In travelling long distances from hospital to hospital, while performing these post-mortems, a bottle of absolute formalin (40 per cent.) could be easily carried in my pocket and diluted with water as occasion required. The liability of formalin to precipitate haemoglobin in granular form in the tissues under tropical conditions is another disadvantage which it possesses as a fixative.

(2) *A description of the morbid anatomy of sprue as met with in Ceylon*

Macroscopic. I have based my description of the morbid anatomy of sprue on two post-mortems of Europeans. I do not propose to enter in this place into details; these are related in full in Appendices XI and XII where the weights of the various organs are also given. The microscopic findings have been confirmed in part by sections obtained from four native cases.

The post-mortems were made under the most favourable circumstances within two hours of death, thus reducing to a minimum the liability to rapid post-mortem decomposition and autodigestion of the abdominal organs, so liable, in the absence of any refrigerating apparatus, to occur in the hot and damp atmosphere of Colombo.

The bodies presented the external appearance of starvation. There was a complete absence of subcutaneous and body fat. The muscles were dark brown in colour, the heart was small, dark brown and atrophied. In fact all the organs were wasted, most of them being less than half the normal weight; this was especially the case with the liver (25 ozs.), and spleen (1½ ozs.) (*vide* Appendix XII). The liver was yellow, friable and fatty (bile-stained in one case), the gall bladder was full of normal-looking bile.

There was a complete absence of fat in the great and small omenta and appendices epiploicae. On opening the abdomen the most noticeable feature was the transparent and distended condition of the ileum. No intestinal ulceration was found (though small superficial follicular ulcers were found in one native case in the large intestine). The

PLATE III

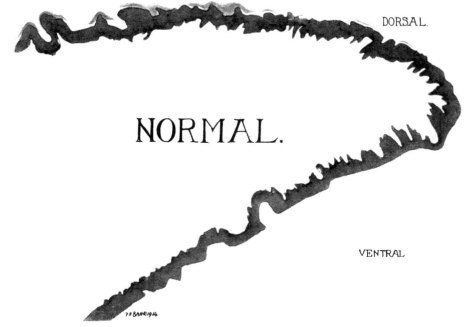

DORSAL.

NORMAL.

VENTRAL

Fig. 1.

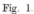

DORSAL

SPRUE.

VENTRAL

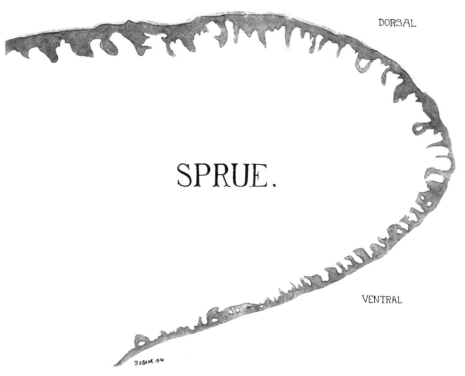

Fig. 2.

Longitudinal mesial sections through the tip of the tongue showing the epithelial covering in

Fig. 1   a normal tongue,   Fig. 2   a sprue tongue.

(Both of these figures are drawn to the same scale with the aid of a camera lucida.)

whole of the intestinal canal was covered with a layer of ropy mucus. The tongue was covered with a film of thrush, only the bases of the fungiform papillae could be distinguished, though on the posterior portion the circumvallate papillae appeared to be intact. The oesophagus in both cases was covered with a yellowish substance, resembling a diphtheritic membrane, which was composed almost entirely of yeast fungus. No gross lesions were detected in any of the viscera.

Microscopic. The red bone marrow was dark in colour and exhibited no peculiar features. In smears made from the liver of post-mortem B a few yeast cells were found, but not in preparations from the other organs.

Numerous cultures were made from all the organs. Yeasts were grown in glucose-broth from every part of the intestinal canal, also in one case from the liver and spleen, and from the kidneys in the other. Cultures from the heart's blood in the first of these yielded a plentiful growth of *Bacillus coli*, apparently of two varieties. One variety gave the typical reactions of the colon bacillus and was toxic to guinea-pigs (2 c.c. intraperitoneally); the other produced no clot in milk and was non-toxic to guineapigs. Similar bacilli were isolated from the mucus of the intestinal canal. I see no reason for incriminating either of these colon bacilli as being concerned in the aetiology of this disease; they most probably denote a secondary, or a terminal infection.

In the microscopic pathology, the points of importance are the desquamation of the stratified surface epithelium of the tongue (Plate III, figs. 1 and 2) and oesophagus, the infiltration of the dead and desquamated and, in some instances, actually of the apparently living and functioning cells by oval yeasts and by a branching mycelium which, in some instances, can be traced growing vertically downwards into the deeper layers (Plates IV and V). As far as one can judge from sections, no such invasion of the mucosa of the stomach or small intestine has taken place, though an occasional budding yeast cell can be seen within the mucosa.

Preparations of the intestinal mucus, stained by Weigert, show an extraordinary number of yeast cells and branching mycelia; in fact these are by far the most abundant organisms present (Plate VII, fig. 1).

It is curious that Justi, though in his post-mortem he observed "oidium-like" threads in the tongue cells and the oesophagus, does not lay much stress on the observation, but incriminates a Gram-positive bacillus he found in the superficial epithelial cells. In all my sections of the tongue and oesophagus bacteria were absent in the deeper tissue layers and were only found in the desquamated and evidently dead epithelial débris.

In addition to this abundant growth of yeast cells in the mucus, several petechial spots were found on minute examination in the walls of the oesophagus and stomach. In scrapings made with a fine needle, threads of branching mycelium and yeast cells evidently growing into the submucosa were found. I did not succeed in making a microscopical section through such a lesion.

DESCRIPTION OF PLATE IV

Fig. 1.   Section of sprue tongue shown in Pl. I, fig. 9, stained by the Weigert-Gram method, showing denudation of surface epithelium; (A) penetration of mycelial threads; (B) granules, probably keratohyaline; (C) Russell's bodies. × 345.

Fig. 2.   Section of sprue spleen stained by Weigert's method, showing (A) Gram-positive bodies in the endothelial cells of the veins; (B) Russell's bodies among the pulp cells; (C) red-blood corpuscles. × 800.

Fig. 3.   Section of sprue tongue through a fungiform papilla: (1) a colony of *Monilia albicans*, (2) penetrating mycelium, (3) degenerating nucleus of epithelial cell, (4) collection of polymorphonuclear leucocytes among dead epithelial cells, (5) desquamating epithelial cells, (6) dilated capillary, (7) plasma cell, (8) apex of fungiform papilla stripped of epithelium, (9) fibroblast, (10) lymphocyte. × 670.

Fig. 4.   Scraping from a sore patch on a sprue tongue showing invasion of epithelial cell by yeast cells; (N) nucleus of epithelial cell, (Y) yeast cells. Stained by eosin-azur. × 1500.

Great interest centres in the microscopical lesions found in the intestinal canal. Sections of the stomach appear normal, but the part of the intestinal canal from duodenum to rectum exhibits changes indicative of a chronic inflammation. In the small intestine the villi are quadrangular in shape and shrunken, the columnar surface epithelium is for the most part preserved[1], but the cells stain badly and the nuclei can with difficulty be distinguished. Chronic inflammatory changes are evident; the capillaries are congested and the interstitial tissue is packed with small round cells and larger cells (leucocytes and plasma cells); the vessels of the submucosa are greatly dilated; there is a

---

[1] This statement is in direct opposition to all the more generally accepted views of the pathology of sprue, but in agreement with the figures and descriptions of Faber and Justi. It is possible that in my cases a limited amount of epithelial destruction took place after death and it is also possible that in such a chronic disease in which the terminal phase is so prolonged (in one case the patient was comatose for ten days before death) a certain amount of destruction of the glandular structures takes place during the last few days of life. It must be remembered in this connection that Bloch in his careful studies found that destruction of columnar epithelium had taken place in those of his experimental animals in which the death agony had been prolonged.

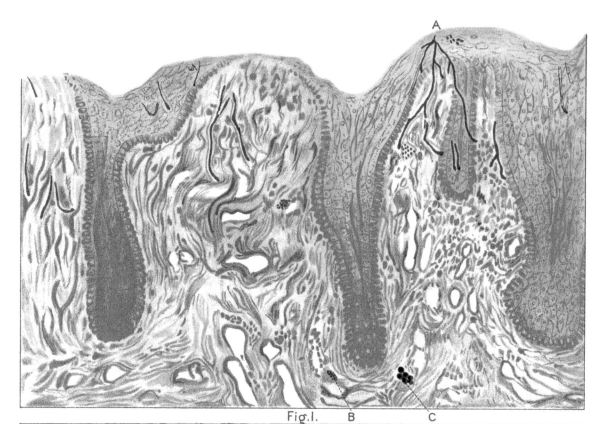

Fig.1.

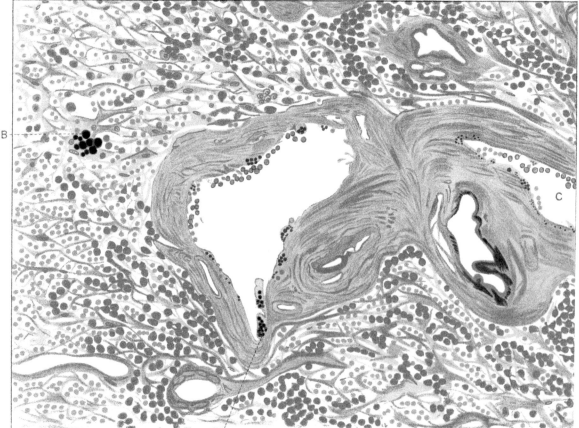

P.H.Bahr del.

Fig.2.

PLATE IV.

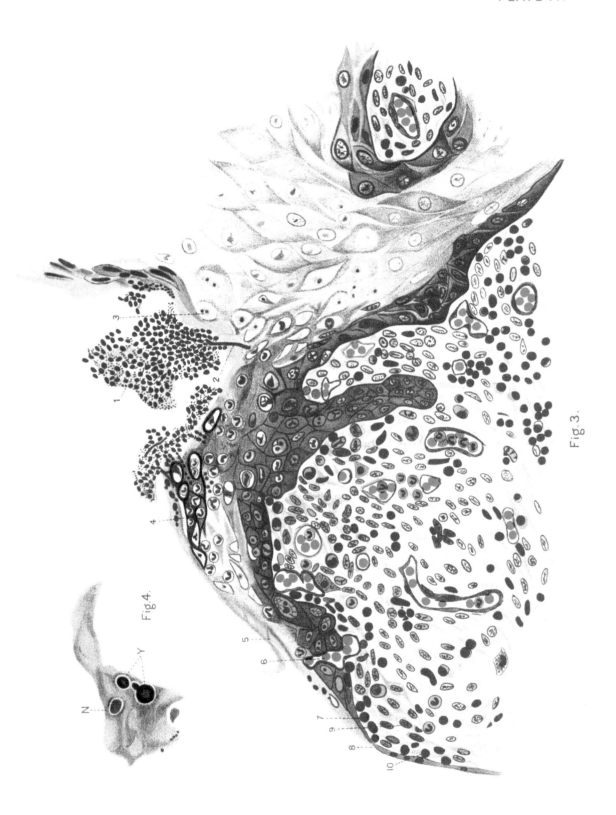

Fig. 3.

Fig. 4.

Cambridge University Press.

general fibrosis and the goblet cells at the fundus of Lieberkühn's crypts are distended (Plate VI). Leucocytes are seen invading the crypts and lying between the secreting cells. In thionin stained sections numerous organisms are seen in the lumen of the crypts and also in the surface columnar epithelial cells. There is some evidence that the muscular coats have been affected by the same inflammatory condition.

Of the other organs examined the condition of two only calls for special attention, namely the liver and spleen. The parenchyma cells of the liver have undergone fatty degeneration at the periphery of the lobules and contain numerous granules of haemosiderin[1] and a few granules of bile pigment. The larger bile ducts are full of Gram-positive bacilli and streptococci, indicating probably a terminal ascending infection of the gall bladder and hepatic ducts by these organisms. In the spleen there are certain changes of evidently a degenerative nature which I believe (and I have endeavoured, as will be gathered, to control my work in every way) to be a hyaline degeneration characteristic of the disease (Plate IV, fig. 2). In the trabecular fibrous tissue there are to be seen large and dilated venules, the swollen endothelial cells of which are packed with round Gram-positive bodies—evidently of a hyaline nature—which distend the cell to bursting point. The nuclei of the cells affected are either absent or are degenerated. With Giemsa these hyaline spheres take on a pink or purple colour, but unlike Russell's bodies, which I will shortly refer to, they are not acid fast to fuchsin, though strongly eosinophile. These bodies were found in every sprue spleen, six in all, of which I obtained sections.

The spherical bodies are of varying sizes; this, together with the absence of any differentiation in their structure, and the lack of surrounding tissue reaction, tend to negative a parasitic origin, favouring rather the idea that they represent some form of cellular degeneration. If such be the explanation, this degeneration must not be confused with another type known as Russell's bodies which are also commonly found in sprue tissues. Russell's bodies are comparatively large hyaline spheres of varying sizes, sometimes small and occurring in clumps or chains, at other times large and solitary; they are markedly Gram-positive and, in contradistinction to the bodies in the splenic capillary endothelium, are feebly acid fast.

[1] Haemosiderin granules, or granules of a pigment resembling haemosiderin, are found in the heart muscle, in the splenic pulp and in the renal epithelial cells of six sprue post-mortems. The iron reaction which was obtained in the case of the liver and spleen is by no means so marked either in bulk or as seen in microscopical sections as in the pernicious anaemia tissues with which I have compared it.

" Russell's bodies."

Special interest attaches to these so-called Russell's bodies which were first described as "cancer bodies," or Russell's fuchsin bodies, and have often subsequently been supposed to be parasites and the cause of tumour growths. As already stated they are hyaline spherical bodies of varying size, the mean being that of a red blood corpuscle. They are found lying singly or in groups, attached to each other, both intracellularly and free in the stroma. They are Gram-positive and stain intensely red with acid fuchsin. Though common in tumour tissues they are also found in inflammatory conditions and are considered to be examples of a hyaline degeneration, but whether of red corpuscles, of cells or of albuminous matter is still unsettled. Of these bodies Adami writes (Adami and Macrae, *Text-Book of Pathology*, 1913, 312), "the intracellular bodies are of various forms, they may be a single round homogeneous mass pushing the nucleus aside, or such a body with a metachromatic central part, or surrounded by a clear space a peripheral ring staining differently from the rest of the body, or by a peripheral ring with processes connecting it with the cytoplasm, or again a central body may be surrounded by a ring of smaller globules, recalling the successive stages of a protozoon with progressive enlargement and final setting free of spores."

Bodies[1] identical with Russell's bodies are commonly found in sprue tissues, especially in the alimentary canal, in all the six postmortems I obtained. But this is not their only situation, as they were found in the tongue, the mucosa of the oesophagus, of the stomach, the duodenum, the ileum, caecum, sigmoid and rectum, in the heart, pancreas, suprarenals, mesenteric lymphatic glands, bone marrow and among the splenic pulp cells. (Plate IV, fig. 2.)

To determine whether these bodies in the submucosa of the intestines are distinctive of sprue or not, I examined the tissues from thirty-eight other post-mortems from Ceylon. Eight were of chronic diarrhoea simulating sprue, but in whom no ankylostomes were found; twelve were cases of ankylostomiasis with terminal diarrhoea; the remainder were miscellaneous cases of tuberculosis, amoebic desentery, malignant disease, etc. In ankylostomiasis they were present in the mucosa of the duodenum, jejunum and transverse colon; they were found also in an amoebic abscess of the liver, in a lymphosarcomatous gland, in a tubercular gland and intestine, all of which are diseases of a chronic inflammatory nature. They were not found in the intestines or other organs of pernicious anaemia, or in acute inflammatory conditions of the intestinal canal, such as bacillary dysentery (three cases). Neither

---

[1] That is they give the same staining reactions as a typical hyaline degeneration and do not agree with the reactions given for mucoid degeneration (purple with thionin blue), colloid (orange-red with Van Gieson), lardaceous (pink with methyl violet), glycogenic (mahogany-red with Lugol's solution), myelin (soluble in hot alcohol).

PLATE V

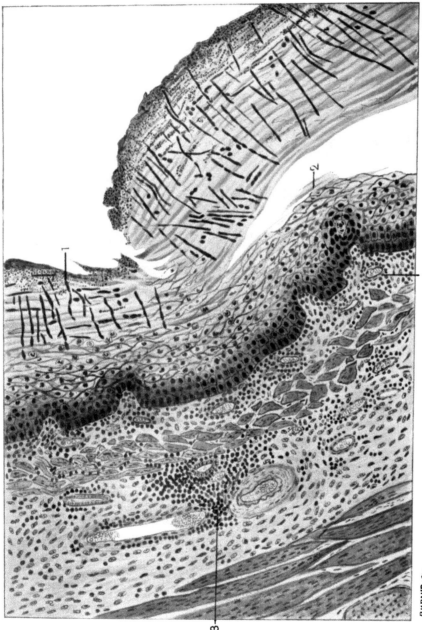

P.H.BAHR 1914.

Section of oesophagus in a case of sprue showing desquamation of stratified epithelium, infiltration of tissues by yeast cells and mycelium, and subacute inflammatory changes in mucous and areolar coats, (1) mycelium penetrating the stratified epithelium in a vertical and horizontal direction, (2) desquamating stratified epithelium, (3) collection of lymphocytes in the areolar coat, (4) perivascular round cell infiltration. × 400.

when present in the splenic pulp cells are they distinctive of sprue, as similar bodies were found in that situation in three cases of malaria; in four of ankylostomiasis and in two of amoebic dysentery.

Russell's bodies[1] are of still further interest to the tropical pathologist. They appear to be identical with the bodies described and figured by Archibald in a paper "Botryomycosis in the Soudan" (*Wellcome Reports*, vol. A, Med. 1911, 337). These bodies (*Botryomyces ascoformans*, Bollinger, 1869), according to Archibald, resemble huge staphylococci, and are three to twelve in number varying in size from 8–12·8 μ. They retain Gram's stain and are slightly acid fast. In man they were found in slowly growing tumours of the breast, face and scalp, and also in a tumour removed from a camel, but since a streptothrix was also found in association, Archibald believes them to be gonidia of a new and hitherto undescribed species of fungus.

According to Wooldridge (*Syst. of Vet. Surg.* Wallis Hoare, 1913) and Kitt (*Textb. Comp. Path.* 1906) *botryomycosis* is known as a widespread disease of horses, cattle and pigs and occurs as actinomycotic tumours said to be caused by this organism, *Botryomyces ascoformans*, a fungus occurring in blackberry masses (50–100 μ in size) made up of conglomerated round disc-like zoogloea masses of cocci. The organism, it is said, will grow on any of the ordinary media, but that on cultivation it becomes much reduced in size and resembles *Staphylococcus pyogenes aureus*.

My investigations on this subject certainly suggest that the structures called *Botryomyces ascoformans* represent a hyaline degenerative change of the same nature as Russell's bodies found in sprue tissue, and therefore cannot be regarded in any way as representing a parasitic organism.

I have failed to find these bodies in lymphatic tissue infected with the *Actinomyces bovis*, but they cannot be regarded as being invariably associated with chronic inflammatory conditions, since I have failed to find them in every tubercular gland I have examined.

I have next to consider *whether these hyaline Gram-positive, but not acid fast bodies, in the endothelial cells of the spleen represent a degeneration pathognomonic of and peculiar to sprue.*

To determine this point, I have examined the spleen microscopically from forty-three other post-mortems, in none of which did I find a similar degeneration.

In twenty-two of these post-mortems the immediate cause of death was diarrhoea; amongst them were four cases of amoebic dysentery and ten cases of ankylostomiasis, but in the remaining eight the origin of the diarrhoea could not be ascertained.

In addition to these I have examined the spleen microscopically in other diseases in which blood destruction is a prominent feature, such as malaria (three cases), kala-azar (two cases), pernicious anaemia (two cases), ankylostomiasis without

---

[1] Russell's bodies must not be confused with granules of keratohyaline which are of irregular shape and are also Gram-positive. In sprue tongues masses of such granules can be seen in the vacuolated and degenerated epithelial cells.

diarrhoea (two cases), tuberculosis with terminal diarrhoea (three cases), lymphatic and spleno-medullary leucocythaemia (one case each), trypanosomiasis and pellagra (one case each) and a miscellaneous series in which the cause of death was pneumonia, uraemia, lymphosarcoma, filariasis, bacillary dysentery, etc.

I realise that this degeneration may possibly represent an early stage of the typical Russell's bodies from which they can be differentiated only by their small size and by their staining reactions, and that when set free in the blood stream they may agglomerate and assume a different form and chemical composition.

As to their exact nature I have been unable to reach any definite conclusions, but I am inclined to regard them as being possibly a degeneration produced in response to the extensive yeast infection found in sprue. In support of this view I can adduce at least one fact, namely, that bodies giving the same staining reactions were produced in the capillary endothelium of the liver of one rabbit after intravenous injection with yeasts isolated from a sprue saliva. A similar degeneration of the spleen could not, however, by any of these means be produced in other experimental animals.

No pathological changes could be found in the sprue pancreas, on macroscopic, and little, save a fine interalveolar fibrosis on microscopic examination.

I shall now proceed to consider various other points in the pathology of sprue, to which I have already briefly alluded.

(1) *Are the lesions found in the tongue characteristic of sprue ?*

The changes found in sections of the sprue tongues I have examined are briefly as follows:

(*a*) Active desquamation of the surface epithelium.

(*b*) Progressive degeneration of the deeper epithelial layer, as evidenced by vacuolation of the cells, degeneration of their nuclei and local aggregations of leucocytes.

(*c*) Inflammatory changes in the corium of the papillae.

(*d*) Infiltration of the surface epithelium and corium of the papillae by mycelium and oval yeast cells (in four out of the six sprue tongues sectionised).

To determine whether these changes can be considered at all pathognomonic of the sprue tongue, I have examined the tongues

PLATE VI

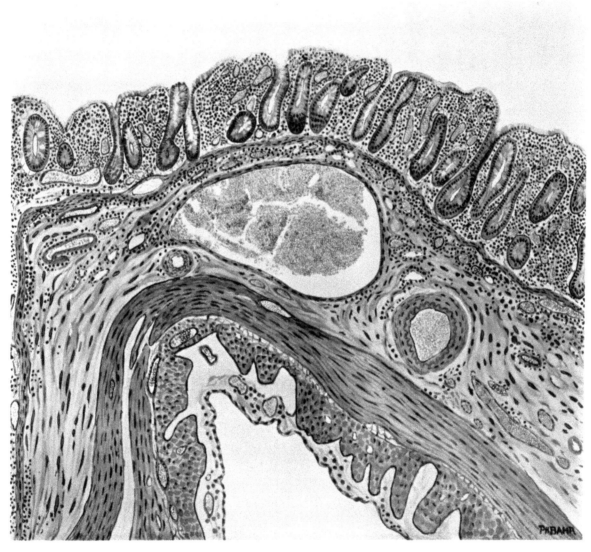

Section of ileum in a case of sprue showing presence of surface epithelium, distension of the goblet cells, atrophy of the villi, infiltration with inflammatory cells, fibrosis of the submucosa, slight perivascular round cell infiltration, great capillary congestion.   × 200.

(Reproduced by permission of the Society of Tropical Medicine and Hygiene.)

from thirty-four other cases in the majority of which there was a terminal diarrhoea, such as ankylostomiasis, amoebic and bacillary dysentery, tubercular enteritis and a case of pernicious anaemia. In only one out of this large series were all the lingual papillae atrophied; this was a specimen taken from a year old Indian child who had suffered from thrush during life. In a section of this tongue the microscopic changes already described in sprue were present even to the superficial penetration of the surface epithelium by yeast cells and mycelium.

In five tongues of the control series the dead epithelium on the summit of the papillae was infiltrated with yeast cells, but the underlying cells appeared perfectly normal; no penetration of mycelial threads into the deeper layers of the tongue could be seen, thereby suggesting a non-pathogenic saprophytic habit of the fungus in these cases.

In the pernicious anaemia tongue the epithelial layer was much attenuated and the cells appeared to be degenerating, thus representing possibly a nutritional change.

In sections of a tongue from a case of "tongue sprue" (Appendix XI, post-mortem G), the same desquamation of the epithelial cells and yeast invasion are present as in the sprue tongues. I have already noted (Chapter XII) that the symptoms presented during life by cases of this description seem to have a definite connection with those of genuine sprue; the similarity in the microscopical lesions of the tongue therefore lends additional colour to this view.

As far as the evidence I have brought forward on the subject goes, we may conclude that there is no essential difference between the microscopical structure of the sprue tongue and that of the infant's tongue affected in a similar manner by the thrush fungus.

(2) *Are the lesions found in the alimentary canal characteristic of sprue?*

(a) *Oesophagus.* I have been unable in any specimens collected in Ceylon to find the marked desquamation of the epithelial cells and infiltration with yeast fungi in this organ as in the sprue oesophagus, but through the kindness of Dr Hubert Turnbull of the London Hospital, I was enabled to examine the tissues of a child dead of chronic diarrhoea and in whom the oesophagus was covered with an anginal membrane composed entirely of yeast cells and mycelial elements which have caused complete destruction of the mucous layer and have penetrated the muscularis mucosae, and were actually found in small ulcerations of the colon[1]. Similar pseudo-anginal membranes of the oesophagus caused by the thrush fungus have been reported from time to time in temperate zones in subjects of chronic wasting disease by Parrot, Brandenberg, Herzfeld and Langerhans.

(b) *Stomach.* A degree of round cell infiltration in the mucosa was the only abnormal change noted in the sprue stomach, but this feature cannot in any way be considered characteristic of the disease, for I have found a more marked degree of round cell infiltration in many ankylostomiasis cases and especially in pernicious anaemia. Whether such a condition really represents a chronic inflammatory change is open to doubt, for, as has been pointed out by Faber, it is probably partly dependent on the degree of functional activity of this organ at the time of death.

(c) *Duodenum and jejunum.* The round cell infiltration of the mucosa and the chronic inflammatory changes in the submucosa are certainly more marked in sprue than in any of the control tissues, including many cases of ankylostomiasis, which I have examined.

(d) *Ileum. Is the transparency and apparent thinning of the ileum characteristic of sprue?*

I performed a number of post-mortems (thirty-seven in all) on cases of chronic diarrhoea in natives in order to ascertain whether a similar condition of the ileum could be found. I roughly estimated the transparency of the gut according to the degree I was able to read print through it. I found no less than nine cases in which a similar degree of transparency was found. In all of these the degree of anaemia was extreme; in five great numbers of ankylostome worms were found in the small intestine[2]; in the remaining four there was no such specific exciting cause of the anaemia. I also have been able by the kind permission of Dr H. B. Newham to examine the intestinal canal in a case of pernicious anaemia, in this latter instance also a similar degree of transparency was present.

Since in none of these nine cases could the transparency be ascribed to the actual loss of any tissue in the bowel wall I am forced to conclude

---

[1] There are other points in this case which are of interest in this connection. The child was eight months old, and suffered from diarrhoea and vomiting since six weeks of age. At the post-mortem the *lingual papillae were atrophied*; there was a granular greyish-white membrane covering the pharynx and part of the oesophagus, mucous catarrh of the whole of the intestinal tract and lenticular ulceration of the splenic flexure of the colon; wasting was extreme.

[2] According to Dr R. T. Leiper *Necator americanus* is by far the most abundant species of ankylostome amongst the specimens I preserved.

that the apparent thinning of the ileum in sprue is due, partly to the distension of the gut wall by the gaseous contents, and partly to its anaemic condition.

Most authors have laid special stress on this thinning of the ileum as being a striking, if not a pathognomonic feature of sprue. As a result of my work, I am unable to support this view, for I find on actual measurement of my microscopical sections that the sprue sections compare favourably in actual thickness of the bowel with the controls.

I have been forced, therefore, to conclude that there is no more evidence for regarding the loss of surface epithelium and the attenuation of the gut as being any more characteristic of sprue than it is of any other diarrhoea.

I have now to consider whether the characteristic shape of the villi and the marked inflammatory changes of the mucosa can be considered characteristic of the disease.

In all cases of chronic diarrhoea there are necessarily evidences of chronic irritation of the gut wall, such as round cell infiltration of the mucosa and capillary dilatation. These changes are present in varying degrees of severity in all the cases I have mentioned. On the other hand, I have been unable to find in any case a similar degree of fibrosis of the submucosa, or such a marked congestion of the nutrient vessels of the submucosa as I found in sprue.

(e) *Large intestine*. What I have already stated with regard to the small intestine applies with equal force to the large. In sprue post-mortem B I found localised transparent patches in the caecum, but no change in any other portion of the intestinal canal; in post-mortem A, this feature was absent. In no case of chronic diarrhoea did I discover a similar attenuation of any part of the large intestine.

In no single control case, uncomplicated by ulceration, were the chronic inflammatory changes in the mucosa, and which extended into the rectum itself, so well marked as in sprue.

(f) *Bone marrow*. I have compared, both in smears and in sections, the structure of the bone marrow in sprue with similar preparations from a case of pernicious anaemia.

Apart from the atrophy of the fat cells in the sprue bone marrow, I can find nothing abnormal, such as an increase in the normoblastic elements which is described in pernicious anaemia.

There is then no evidence, from the small amount of work I was able to do on this subject, of any specific affection of the blood-forming tissues in sprue as there is in pernicious anaemia.

I append a table for comparison of the pathology of sprue and pernicious anaemia, the former based upon my pathological findings in Ceylon, the latter upon the more recently accepted descriptions of the latter disease. Such a table I have deemed it advisable to insert, seeing that the two diseases have undoubtedly certain features in common and seeing that authorities are inclined to regard an intestinal toxaemia as being the chief aetiological factor in the pathology of the latter disease also.

	Pernicious anaemia	*Sprue*
Body	Not specially wasted; lemon-yellow subcutaneous and tissue fat present.	Wasting extreme; fat absent.
Muscles	Not wasted, bright pink in colour.	Wasted, dark brown in colour.
Serous surfaces	Patchy haemorrhages often present.	Absent usually.
Heart	Fatty and enlarged (tabby-cat striation).	Dark brown and cardiac cells atrophied (brown atrophy).
Liver	Large and fatty; iron reaction well marked.	Small and fatty; iron reaction present, but not so marked.
Spleen	Size variable, generally enlarged; iron reaction well marked.	Small and atrophied; iron reaction present, but not so marked.
Red marrow	Bright red in colour, characteristic microscopical changes.	Dark red in colour; microscopically no increase of erythroblastic elements.
Intestinal mucus	Apparently not increased in amount.	Increased in amount.
Microscopical structure of intestines	Round cell infiltration sometimes present (Hunter).	Round cell infiltration marked.
Russell's bodies	Not found (two cases).	Common in alimentary mucosa, spleen, heart, etc.
Hyaline degeneration of venous endothelium of spleen	Absent.	Present.
General yeast infection	Absent.	Present.

For comparison of actual weights of organs see Appendix XII.

CHAPTER XV

THE AETIOLOGY OF SPRUE

THEORIES in numbers have been put forward as to the cause of sprue. These may be divided and discussed under three headings: (a) climatic, (b) dietetic, (c) specific.

(a) *Climatic theory.* Mainly on the ground of its distribution and of its apparent limitation to individuals of European origin, some observers have been inclined to regard sprue as being a non-specific disease, or as some disorder of metabolism occasioned by the unaccustomed climatic conditions.

Bosch, Van der Burg and Manson inclined to the view that the hyperactivity of the digestive organs occasioned by tropical conditions ends in exhaustion and apepsia and thus induces the symptoms and pathological lesions peculiar to sprue.

I have already dealt with this question and have given my reasons for disregarding the climate as being other than a predisposing factor.

(b) *Dietetic theory.* The highly-spiced foodstuffs peculiar to the East have also been inculpated. For instance Schneider, who practised thirty years in Java, regarded the diminution in the number of cases coming under his observation as being the direct result of the diminished use of such condiments. Cantlie has incriminated the oils used in cooking in the tropics.

I have already stated my views on these points.

(c) *Specific theory.* It must be admitted that little positive evidence has been so far brought forward in support of any specific organism as being the cause of sprue, but for the convenience of description, I have subdivided such evidence as there is into three headings: the verminous, bacillary and fungoid.

Verminous infection. There is little to be said in support of a helminthic infection.

In 1877 Normand regarded the *Anguillula intestinalis*, so common in certain parts of the East, as the cause of the Cochin-China diarrhoea;

later observers, however, showed that the *Anguillula* is a parasite of common occurrence in the East and in no way essentially associated with sprue.

Bacillary infection. It cannot be said that the bacterial theory of sprue has much to recommend it.

The tropical distribution, if not limitation, of sprue is not in accordance with the distribution of any known bacterial disease.

Thin isolated a number of micro-organisms from the stools, but was unable to bring forward any convincing proof of their specific nature. He also remarked on the apparent scarcity of *B. coli* in sprue stools.

Goadby has isolated Flexner's dysentery bacillus from sprue stools. Castellani[1] has described a similar organism from cases presenting sprue-like symptoms. Musgrave has isolated *B. coli* in pure culture from the heart's blood, but it is open to doubt as to whether this was the result of a secondary infection or not (*vide* post-mortem B, Appendix XI). Faber in a post-mortem performed in Copenhagen found a diplococcus in the intestinal mucus, in the peritoneal exudate and in the heart's blood; this organism was non-pathogenic to guineapigs.

Justi (Dec. 1913) suspects a Gram-positive bacillus which he found in the tissues and which has been successfully cultivated by Beneke and Ungermann, but so far no further experimental work has been published on this subject.

It is possible that the preponderance of any species of bacillus in the sprue stools is dependent on certain chemical changes in the bowel contents; the latter being themselves the result of pathological changes in the digestive glands. Further we know from the researches of Lembke[2] and others[3] that the bacterial flora— especially the preponderance of *B. coli* and the chemical composition of the stool— varies with different diets. It appears that with the use of new ingredients in a diet the numbers of *B. coli* become fewer but that it becomes prevalent once more after it has had time to accommodate itself to the new conditions.

I examined a series of nine sprue stools in order to ascertain the number of *B. coli* colonies present. These specimens were plated

---

[1] Castellani (*Journ. Trop. Med. and Hyg.* 1912, p. 337) isolated a "Flexner-like" bacillus from three cases of "pseudo-sprue," whose sera agglutinated the organisms. My experience of the symptoms of sprue leads me to believe that the cases described by the author are merely aberrant forms of the typical disease; indeed I believe one of the cases which he quotes in his paper died shortly after my arrival in the Colony, apparently with all the symptoms typical of sprue.

[2] Lembke (1896), *Archiv f. Hyg.* XXVI, 325.

[3] Tissier (1908), *Annal. Inst. Past.* 187; Escherich (1886), *Die Darmbakterien des Säuglings*, Stuttgart, 112.

out on neutral-red agar. In some instances colonies of *B. coli* were extremely rare in proportion to those of other bacteria—1-15; in other instances they were found to be two and a half times as numerous as all the other bacteria together.

From the mucus surrounding one sprue stool I isolated a dysentery-like organism almost in pure culture. That is to say it was a non-motile, Gram-negative bacillus, and gave similar reactions in solutions of the sugars in peptone water (it produced acid in mannite, dextrose and maltose but not in saccharose). Even in its milk reactions it resembled the dysentery organism, but it was not agglutinated by a polyvalent antidysenteric nor the patient's serum. It was non-pathogenic to guineapigs and a culture injected into the intestinal canal of rabbits produced no symptoms.

A Gram-positive diplococcus was cultivated from the sprue stools in four and from the saliva in seven instances. I attached little importance to their presence for after long subculture some of the strains assumed streptococcal form (probably *Streptococcus faecalis* and *Streptococcus brevis* respectively).

In centrifuged extracts of some sprue stools I certainly noted an undue preponderance of Gram-positive bacilli. It is possible that the abnormal composition of the sprue stool may also account for their prevalence.

Fungoid infection. In 1901 Kohlbrugge found in the intestinal mucus, in the lymphoid patches of the intestinal canal, and in the epithelial covering of the tongue and oesophagus, great quantities of yeast cells resembling *Monilia (oidium) albicans*. These organisms grew equally as well on acid as on alkaline media. A similar organism was found in the faeces of other patients not suffering from sprue.

In 1902 De Haan found these organisms only in the acid, but not in the alkaline sprue stools. On these grounds he considered that they played no part in the aetiology of the disease.

In 1905 Van der Scheer reported his inability to find these organisms in scrapings of the inflamed sprue tongue or in the gastric contents in two cases.

In 1908 Le Dantec described a yeast in the stools with an especial affinity for iodine and claimed that with cultures of this organism he was able to produce sprue symptoms in experimental animals, if once a diarrhoea had been established by some other means.

In 1909 Macy, at the Bombay Medical Congress, described a similar yeast as occurring in sprue stools in India.

Castellani and Low in 1913 (*Journ. Trop. Med.* 1913, 34) have described a number of species of yeast (as differentiated by their sugar reactions), which they isolated from sprue stools, but neither of these observers regards this as otherwise than a secondary infection with the thrush fungus, though they think it possible that it plays a part in the production of the frothy stools. They consider that sprue is really a communicable protozoal disease.

In addition to having described a dysentery bacillus and various species ·of yeast as being associated with sprue lesions Castellani (1912) (*Journ. Trop. Med.* 354) has further noted a clamydozoon-like body which he has found in the tongue epithelium. His preparations were derived from a European woman whom I saw on my arrival in Colombo and on whom a year afterwards I performed an autopsy (post-mortem A, Appendix XI). I have failed, either in scrapings made during life or in sections of the organ post-mortem, to find any structures similar to the bodies described by Castellani. In this, as well as in other cases of sprue, some ill-defined granular masses can certainly be demonstrated in the epithelial cells in preparations stained by haematoxylin, carbol gentian violet and by eosin-azure, but similar bodies were found in normal tongues. They most probably represent a stage in the degeneration of the cell protoplasm.

In passing it is interesting to note that this investigator has also described other organisms in sprue; he has noted (*Manual of Tropical Medicine* (1913), 2nd ed. 1327) a "*spirochaete or treponema-like germ*" (site not mentioned), and peculiar bodies in the lymphocytes and polymorphonuclear cells of the blood resembling the bodies of E. H. Ross in syphilis.

Appendicitis. It is only necessary to refer shortly to the theory put forward by Van der Scheer. This observer found unmistakable signs of inflammation of the vermiform appendix in thirty cases of sprue, in several instances improvement after operation was noted.

Significance of yeasts in sprue

I have already alluded to the vastness of the numbers of yeast cells and mycelia found in tongue scrapings and in the oesophageal and intestinal mucus in my sprue post-mortems. As similar organisms could be cultivated from the internal organs—spleen (one case), kidneys and liver—it might be thought that there was at least some evidence of a general blastomycotic infection in sprue and, possibly, of an aetiological relationship of a yeast fungus to the disease.

As regards the evidence in favour of such a hypothesis afforded by the circumstance that I succeeded in cultivating yeasts from the tissues referred to I must confess that little weight can be attached to it; for although cultures revealed the presence of yeasts in the tissues direct microscopic investigation of sections failed, or almost failed to do so. It is therefore extremely improbable that so feeble an invasion has any serious bearing on the causation or on the symptoms of sprue.

It is otherwise I think with regard to the enormous mycotic development in the contents of the alimentary canal and it seems to me that the profusion of yeasts in the gut is not without significance, possibly aetiological significance. I therefore propose to consider the subject in some detail.

If the yeasts in sprue are but a secondary or terminal infection a similar invasion of the intestinal mucus should be found in other chronic wasting diarrhoeas, so common in natives. I therefore made cultures and microscopical preparations of the intestinal mucus in every post-mortem I obtained. For many reasons I could place little reliance on the cultural method as indicating such a preponderance of yeast cells in the intestinal canal, but in smears of the intestinal mucus and other organs stained by Gram I was quite unable to find such a heavy infection of the lower intestinal tract with these organisms as I did in sprue, though in some a few yeast cells scattered through the preparations could be seen (*vide* Appendix XIII). In about a third of the cases (nine out of twenty-four), yeast cells could be seen in scrapings of the tongue, and in a similar number they were present also in scrapings of the oesophagus and stomach, but in only one—a case of ankylostomiasis—were a few mycelial elements found in these situations such as would indicate a downward growth of the organism into the tissues.

The technique employed in making these cultures was simple. A small portion of the mucus was taken up from the intestinal canal by means of a metal scraper and inoculated into 4 per cent. glucose-broth. The tubes were incubated for forty-eight hours, shaken up and examined for yeast cells with $\frac{1}{6}$ in. lens. In making cultures from solid organs the surface was first seared and a small portion removed from the centre by the same means, or by means of a sterile syringe in the case of the heart. It must be remembered in making any comparison of these cultural results from the intestinal mucus that yeast cells are ubiquitous in the tropics and may gain entrance to the intestinal canal by the mouth and even from the air directly the intestinal tube is opened.

The almost constant association of yeast cells with the lesions of sprue, post-mortem, seemed to indicate some connection between this yeast infection and the disease, but against such a supposition there is abundant evidence that such a general yeast infection is of a more common occurrence in temperate zones than has been supposed.

I have already referred on page 71 to a generalised infection of the alimentary canal by the thrush fungus occurring in this country. This must not be regarded as an isolated instance. Extension of the thrush fungus into the oesophagus and stomach has been reported by Langerhans and Parrot. Schmorl has seen in several exceptional instances the penetration of the mycelial threads into the capillaries and veins, and therefore believes that a general infection with this fungus may occur; thus this investigator and Baginsky have found them in haemorrhagic areas in the kidneys. They have been found in the liver by Grohe, in pneumonic abscesses by

Klemperers and Levy, and in metastatic growths in the lungs and brain by Pineau. I therefore propose to examine in succeeding paragraphs the evidence in favour of associating the thrush fungus with the typical and familiar symptoms and signs of sprue during life.

Evidence of the association of the thrush fungus with the symptoms of sprue during life

(1) *By direct examination of the tongue lesions.* Scrapings of the inflamed areas were made with a sharpened metal scraper and the epithelial débris thus obtained spread on a slide and stained by Gram and in a variety of other ways.

As these inflammatory areas are very evanescent, I deemed it important to pay special attention to those organisms found in such scrapings only during the acute period. Observations such as these could be carried out only in patients whom I could observe daily and were for this reason necessarily limited in number. In three cases, all in the early stages of the disease (two of whom made a good recovery, the third died after a year), I found in such scrapings numerous yeast cells and mycelial elements lying within the epithelial cells. Such organisms were not present in scrapings made simultaneously from such tongue areas as were not inflamed, neither did I subsequently succeed in demonstrating yeast cells or mycelial elements in similar preparations made from the original but now healed spots. (Plate IV, fig. 4.)

I controlled these observations by means of scrapings from ninety-six normal tongues. It is true that in twelve or 12·5 per cent. of these a few extracellular yeast cells were found, but their occurrence and extracellular location suggested a saprophytic rather than a parasitic habit.

In my search for these yeasts I did not neglect other organisms such as mouth bacteria and spirochaetes. Representatives of the common flora of the mouth were found in tongue scrapings, such as *Bacillus maximus*, *Streptococcus brevis*, *Staphylococci*, *Diplococci* and *Sarcinae*.

In cultures of the saliva and tongue many of the commoner mouth organisms were isolated. In scrapings of the tongue made by the Indian-ink method spirochaetes, resembling in their morphology the ordinary mouth spirochaetes, were found in eight cases, but no significance can be attached to their presence in this situation. (In the scrapings of sore tongues from eight native cases I found a curious striated organism of an undetermined nature depicted in Plate VII, fig. 2.)

PLATE VII

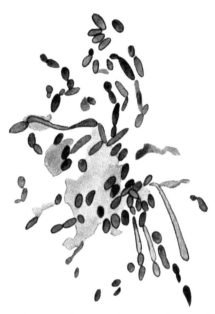

Fig. 1.   Smear prepared from gastric mucus in a case of sprue, showing great numbers
of yeast cells and mycelial threads.   × 1000.

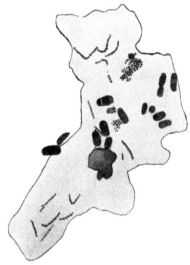

Fig 2.   Curious striated bodies of an undetermined nature found in tongue-scrapings
from eight native cases.   × 1000.

(2) *By culture from the tongue lesions.* Cultures were made from the inflamed tongues by inoculating the scrapings into glucose-broth. In the case of twenty inflamed sprue tongues in Europeans yeast cells were isolated ten times, or in 50 per cent. In the seven fatal cases seen by me immediately before death an abundant growth of these organisms was obtained from the tongue and mouth in every case.

It was necessary to control these observations, as it is obvious that little reliance can be placed on haphazard scrapings from such a septic region as the mouth, a region which cannot be efficiently sterilised.

In scrapings from twenty-three normal European tongues yeast cells were isolated four times, *i.e.* in 17 per cent., but from thirty-two normal native tongues they were obtained ten times, or in 32 per cent.

These observations seem to indicate that the yeast fungus in its downward growth is primarily concerned in the inflammation and ultimate destruction of the lingual papillae and is not to be regarded merely as a secondary epiphenomenon.

(3) *By direct examination of the saliva.* In two cases in which there was no visible deposit of thrush in the mouth, I was surprised to find mycelial threads and yeast cells in abundance in fresh preparations of the saliva. There was no evidence in these cases that the organisms were derived from the bronchi, as they were apparently growing saprophytically in the acid saliva; this acidity probably being due to the growth of the yeast fungus itself, a supposition which I proved to be a possibility by growing these organisms in normal alkaline saliva.

I never again found such a luxuriant growth in the saliva as in these cases, though a few yeast cells could be seen microscopically in ten out of the twenty-four sprue salivas examined.

(4) *By culture of the saliva.* By inducing the patients to expectorate into a glucose-broth tube cultures were made from sprue saliva twenty-nine times. In sixteen, or 55 per cent., yeast cells were isolated. The same objections obviously apply to cultures made in this manner as in the case of the tongue scrapings. In a series of control cases in normal Europeans, yeasts could be isolated by these means in 35 per cent. of the cases.

When these figures[1] are considered in conjunction with other facts

[1] These observations are of importance in another direction. During the last few years Castellani has published several papers on a disease termed by him variously tropical bronchomycosis, bronchoblastomycosis, bronchoendomycosis, bronchoidiosis,

already given I am justified in regarding these organisms as being especially prevalent in sprue saliva.

It would appear that yeast cells may grow abundantly in the saliva even when they cannot be microscopically demonstrated in scrapings of the tongue. Thus in a series of scrapings from eighty-three sore tongues in natives, yeast cells were demonstrated only four times, although in every case they could be cultivated from the saliva.

(5) *By culture from the aphthae.* I have already stated my reasons for disregarding the aphthous ulcerations of the mouth as being essential lesions of sprue. I had great difficulty in obtaining cases in which they were a prominent feature, but I succeeded in examining such aphthous lesions of the tongue and buccal mucous membranes by means of scrapings and cultures in ten instances. In scrapings I could find no organism which I could in any way regard as specific to sprue. *Staphylococci, diplococci* and small *sarcinae* were commonly encountered in the pus cells. In three cases I found yeast cells, but no mycelial elements. *Staphylococcus pyogenes aureus* and *Streptococcus brevis* were commonly isolated on culture. I was unable to differentiate the organisms in the exudate from those found in similar buccal ulcerations in subjects presenting no symptoms of sprue whatsoever. Of these I was able to investigate two cases, one a European planter and the

and bronchomoniliasis. The subjects of this infection are said to exhibit symptoms of subacute or chronic bronchitis, termed "Tea-factory cough," resembling pulmonary tuberculosis; tubercle bacilli, however, cannot be demonstrated in the sputum by microscopical examination, though occasionally numbers of yeast cells can be seen microscopically and can be more frequently isolated by cultural methods. He suggests that the fungi grow saprophytically on tea, since he succeeded in obtaining an abundant growth of these yeasts from specimens of tea examined in Ceylon, but not from specimens of Ceylon tea examined by him in England. He has classified the yeasts obtained from the sputum in these cases into a number of named species.

So far no evidence has been adduced, either post-mortem or in microscopical sections, that such an invasion of the bronchi or lungs by these yeast organisms had, in cases presenting these symptoms, in reality taken place during life.

My observations certainly indicate that these fungi are saprophytic organisms common in the saliva of Europeans in the tropics. It therefore follows that their presence in any given sputum (in which of necessity an admixture of saliva has taken place), does not necessarily denote a pathological bearing.

Certainly none of my sprue patients on whom my observations were made were suffering from "Tea-factory cough" or had any physical signs of disease in their chests.

(References: Castellani (1910), *Phil. Journ. Sci.* 197; (1911), *Journ. Cey. Br. B.M.A.* I.; (1912), *Brit. Med. Journ.* II. 1208; (1912), *Lancet,* I. 13; (1913), *Manual Trop. Med.* 2nd ed. 1284.)

According to the researches of Cao ((1900), *Ztsch. f. Hyg. u. Infektionsk.* XXXIV, 252), yeast cells are especially abundant in tubercular sputum.

other a Sinhalese. It must be remembered that a similar buccal ulceration is commonly found in cachetic children the subjects of a thrush infection, consequently I consider that these lesions are merely the result of a secondary pyogenic infection of a mucous membrane the resistance of which has already been lowered by the cachetic state of the patient or by a primary infection by the thrush fungus.

(6) *By direct examination of the stools.* Special attention was directed to the minute microscopical examination of sprue stools. Those passed by patients under treatment and on a milk diet were selected as being especially suitable and were daily examined over a period of many weeks.

The structures found in the stools of these cases were mainly needles of crystalline fats and soaps. When fruit was added to the diet, the cells characteristic of any particular variety such as the Bael fruit (*Aegle marmelos*), the Pawpaw (*Carica papaya*), the Avocado pear (*Pusea gratissima*) and the Banana could be recognised. As to evidences of protozoal infection, in one case I found numerous flagellates, probably *Trichomonas intestinalis*, and also occasionally in two cases during convalescence, cysts of *Entamoeba coli*; these were probably of adventitious occurrence.

In the frothy acid stools passed during the early stages of the disease, in three cases I saw cells bearing a great resemblance to yeast cells and once short mycelial threads. These cells resemble yeasts in shape and in their affinity for iodine (a property peculiar to the group). From a microscopical examination alone it is almost impossible to decide whether these structures were pure yeasts or organisms identical with *Blastocystis enterocola*, a yeast-like body commonly found in normal stools and whose life history as studied by Alexeieff[1] differs widely from that of the true yeasts.

There is no doubt that yeasts are by far the most predominant organisms in the stools passed shortly before death. I have preserved a smear preparation from such a stool in which this is a most striking feature. I also studied the organisms found in the centrifuged deposit of sprue stools.

The technique was as follows. A small portion of the stool was thoroughly ground up in distilled water and centrifugalised, the resulting deposit was shaken up with absolute alcohol and again centrifuged; smears of the residue were stained by Gram and by a number of other methods.

[1] (1911), *Comp. Rend. de la Soc. de Biol.* LXXI, 269.

By using this method yeast cells, many in the process of division, were found in the deposit of 42 per cent. of sprue stools (fifty-seven in all, from cases of sprue and chronic diarrhoea), but small numbers of similar cells were found in 25 per cent. of normal native and amoebic dysentery stools treated in a similar manner.

Organisms in stools liable to be mistaken for yeast cells. In one sprue stool I found oval organisms corresponding to the figures and descriptions of the *Clostrydium butyricum* of Prazmowski, occurring in chains and possessing a marked affinity for iodine. I did not regard their presence as being of any particular significance.

Sarcinae in packets of four and eight were commonly found and could be cultivated from almost every sprue stool.

Certain small Gram-negative yellow bodies and staining bright blue with eosin-azur, 3–4 μ in length, often possessing a small lateral or terminal excrescence, puzzled me considerably (Plate VIII, fig. 2). I noted, however, that they only appeared in numbers in the stools when either bread or toast formed an essential part of the patients' diet and identical bodies were found in preparations of normal stools. I attempted to cultivate them in welled slides containing glucose-broth and a small amount of stool kept under constant microscopical observation. No development of any sort took place. From their inability to propagate themselves in glucose-broth, and from their shrunken yellow appearance, I concluded that the organisms were dead. I subsequently ascertained that similar bodies could be found in bread and in toast and represented the dead remains of the bakers' yeast which had passed unchanged through the intestinal canal.

(7) *By culture of the stools for yeasts. Technique.* A small portion of the stool, collected in a sterile receptacle, was inoculated by means of a platinum rod into 4 per cent. glucose-broth. It was then incubated for forty-eight hours, shaken up and examined for yeast cells with the $\frac{1}{8}$ in. lens. In order to isolate the organisms in a pure state, the culture was subsequently plated out on glucose-agar.

According to Strasburger, yeast cells may be sparingly cultivated on appropriate media from nearly every normal stool. When one considers that such cells are being constantly ingested in the food, it may be inferred that their presence in the stool in small numbers is of no special significance.

Fifty-nine stools (forty-four from sprue cases and fifteen from cases of chronic diarrhoea) were cultivated in this manner and yeasts were isolated in 55 per cent., whereas they could be cultivated only

PLATE VIII

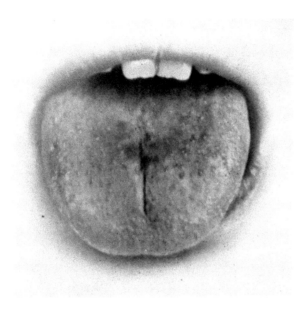

Fig. 1. "Tongue Sprue" in a high-caste Tamil boy.
(Reproduced by permission of the Society of Tropical Medicine and Hygiene.)

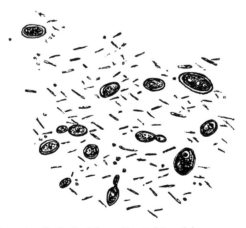

Fig. 2. Dead yeast cells derived from digested bread in a sprue stool. × 1500.

from 29 per cent. of the control cases (normal native, normal European and amoebic dysentery stools).

These figures by no means indicate the excessive prevalence of yeast cells in sprue stools even during the acute stage of the disease. In patients under treatment they could be cultivated in only relatively small numbers after the stools had become solid. An abundant growth of yeasts was invariably obtained from the typical pale and frothy stools.

(8) *Abundance of yeasts in intestinal contents after death.* This point I have already dwelt on. Having previously demonstrated by direct microscopical examination their abundance in the liquid sprue stool removed from the post-mortem table, it was not surprising to find that after plating out such a stool on glucose-agar, and counting the colonies, the yeast colonies were three times as numerous as those of other organisms.

Although it is difficult, in view of the uncertain nature of the whole subject, to draw any definite and positive conclusions, yet I submit that these observations indicate that, not only can yeasts be cultivated from the majority of sprue stools and salivas, but that in the acute, as well as in the terminal stages, they are at least the most prevalent organisms in the tongue lesions, saliva and stools of victims of the disease. I next propose to recount investigations made with the object of ascertaining the identity of the yeast fungi found in sprue lesions during life and post-mortem.

CHAPTER XVI

A STUDY OF THE YEASTS FOUND IN SPRUE LESIONS
AND ATTEMPTS AT THEIR CLASSIFICATION

THE blastomyces, or yeasts, are distinguished from the true fungi by their peculiar mode of reproduction by gemmation. Some kinds, under adverse circumstances, reproduce by means of spores called ascospores or chlamydospores and they can be classified into two main groups: (1) the *Saccharomyces*, and (2) *Torulae*, according to whether these spores are formed or not. Amongst the former of these a third method of growth by the fusion of individual cells to form mycelial threads may also arise, and according to the presence or absence of this mycelium formation the *Saccharomyces* can be further subdivided into two subgroups, the first of which may be termed the *Saccharomyces* proper and the second the *Monilia*, and it is to this latter genus that the thrush fungus belongs.

The thrush fungus. Nomenclature. There has been much confusion in the nomenclature of the thrush fungus. This organism was termed *Oidium albicans* by Langenbeck who discovered it in 1839, and under that name it was referred to by Robin in 1853. In 1899 Vuillemin referred it to the genus *Endomyces* which he created on the supposition that spores were formed within the mycelial threads, an observation which is now held to be incorrect. In 1895 it was renamed *Monilia* by Lydia Rabinowitch who believed it to be identical with the organism named by Gmelin in 1791, therefore, according to the rules of scientific nomenclature, the latter name of the genus has been adopted and the proper scientific name of the thrush fungus has become *Monilia albicans*.

Description. I have been struck with the divergent descriptions of the organism given in most text-books. The following is a summary of these accounts and of my own work on the same subject.

The yeast cells have a definite capsule containing a hyaline plasma with protoplasmic granulations which are by some termed nuclei. According to my observations, in the majority of cells a vacuole containing a minute and rapidly moving body with a marked affinity for iodine can also be distinguished. Individual cells differ markedly in size, but on an average measure 5–6 μ in length by 4 μ in breadth. The cells have a marked affinity for iodine and stain intensely by Gram, though in old cultures this property may be lost; with Rowmanowsky stains a certain amount of ill-defined red-staining material can be made out in the centre of each cell.

Degenerative cells are common in every culture. The mycelium, which is abundantly produced when grown on alkaline media, shows all grades between a true mycelial thread and an agglomeration of three or four actively budding cells; it contains inclusions, granules and vacuoles; it is doubtful, as I have already mentioned, whether spore formation within its substance takes place or not.

Round spore-like structures (ascospores or chlamydospores), of a larger size than the vegetative cells, are budded off from the mycelium. They have a thick capsule and contain a number of granular bodies which, according to some investigators, are capable of regenerating into budding yeasts, but according to others represent merely a degenerative change. The fungus is readily cultivated on the ordinary media especially on those containing a proportion of certain sugars (glucose, maltose and lactose), and produces white slimy adherent growth, though the exact colour may vary on different media.

On slab cultures in gelatin it produces a small amount of liquefaction (probably not a true liquefaction but merely a softening of the medium). On agar plate cultures it occurs in two forms, firstly as round wax-like granulated superficial colonies, secondly as deeper lying colonies with irregularly branched borders. When the medium is dry this branching is exaggerated. An acid medium encourages the growth of vegetative cells, an alkaline one the growth of mycelium.

The carbohydrates are fermented in a variable manner with the production of a certain amount of alcohol, but not in any large quantity as in the case of the *Saccharomyces*. In milk no acidity or clot is produced. The pathogenicity of the fungus has been extensively studied by Cao (1900), *Zeitsch. f. Hyg. u. Infectionsk.* Subcutaneous inoculations in rabbits produced localised abscesses; intraperitoneal inoculations localised mesenteric growths. The results of intravenous injection differed widely; as a rule rabbits died in uraemic convulsions and post-mortem the cortical tissue of the kidneys was found studded with miliary abscesses containing yeast cells and mycelium. These organisms could be isolated from most of the organs and, in some instances, also from the brain. He also investigated identical, if not closely allied, organisms obtained from milk, air, fruit, faeces, etc.;

some of these had a high degree of pathogenicity to rabbits, others none at all.

Lately an attempt has been made, especially by Castellani, to classify these yeasts belonging to the genus *Monilia* into a large number of species according to their reactions with solutions of the different sugars. A brief study of Castellani's classification of this group (*Manual Trop. Med.* (1913), 2nd ed., 822) shows that specific distinctions have been founded in many instances upon very minor variations in these reactions.

In my attempts to classify the yeast fungi found in sprue and in order to compare them with other yeasts, I examined 112 cultures obtained in Ceylon from various sources. Five were cultivated from thrush lesions in infants, and were compared with others obtained from the mouths, stools and post-mortem tissues of sprue cases, and also with cultures obtained from the air, from cowdung, from fruit, milk and from bakers' yeast. According to the classification I have already given, out of these 112 cultures only four could be classified as true *Saccharomyces* and two as true *Torulae*, the remaining 106 belonged to the genus *Monilia* (that is, under certain circumstances they produced an abundant mycelial growth).

Technique of isolation. This has already been given; it is only necessary to state further that all cultures were plated out at regular intervals on glucose-agar so as to avoid bacterial contamination to which such cultures appear to be especially liable.

An attempt was made to classify these 106 *Monilia* strains according to certain features such as

(1) The appearance of the growth.
(2) The size and shape of the vegetative cells.
(3) The tendency to mycelium formation.
(4) The pathogenic action on experimental animals.
(5) The reactions with solutions of various sugars.

As a result of extensive investigations on all these lines I was unable to arrive at any satisfactory basis of classification, as I shall relate.

(1) *Appearance of the growth on culture*

All the strains investigated formed a thick cream-coloured growth on glucose-agar. Minor variations in the appearance of this growth were noted; in many the surface had a dull appearance; in others again it exhibited branching processes extending both laterally and downwards into the substance of the medium. Such minor characters were found to be inconstant on further subculture. Subsequent observations indicated that they depended, not on any inherent character of the fungus, but probably on the exact composition and dryness of the medium employed at the time. When grown anäerobically no difference in the luxuriance or appearance of the growth could be detected. No liquefaction in gelatin stab cultures was produced by any of the organisms investigated; at the most a certain amount of softening of the upper layers of the medium occurred. On alkaline-agar the growth was as luxuriant as on an acid medium.

(2) *The size and shape of the vegetative cells*

A large number of yeast cells in glucose-broth cultures were examined and measured. I had hoped to classify the different cultures by the shape of the individual cells; certain strains were found in which the majority of the cells were either round or elliptical; but even this feature was found to be inconstant on further subculture. With regard to size, individual cells in the same culture varied greatly from 3 to 9 μ in diameter. In some cultures the majority of the cells were of a large size, but even this feature could not be relied upon and depended probably on the virility and the age of the particular culture employed.

(3) *The production of mycelium*

The rapidity and extent to which mycelial threads were formed in cultures varied enormously. It was found that on agar slants the bulk of the mycelium developed in the water of condensation, rarely on the surface growth. Many strains, however, failed to grow any mycelium on solid media, but readily did so in broth cultures. There were other cases in which it was produced only after constant culture for three or more weeks and when presumably the conditions had become unfavourable to reproduction by other methods. The extremes in the rapidity with which this mycelial growth was produced varied in different cultures from a period of twenty-four hours to one of twenty-eight days continuous incubation. This proclivity to mycelium formation even varied greatly in a culture from the same source when tested on several occasions. It may be stated that as a general rule mycelial threads appeared with greater rapidity and in greater numbers on an alkaline (− 10 Eyre's scale) rather than on acid medium.

(4) *The pathogenic action on experimental animals*

Feeding experiments with cultures of sprue yeasts and those of the true *Monilia albicans* produced no ill effects in any animals, even though monkeys and rabbits were fed daily with large doses.

Subcutaneous injections produced localised abscesses in guineapigs; in the resulting pus many vacuolated and evidently defunct yeast cells could be seen microscopically.

Intraperitoneal injections of broth cultures differed widely in their effects. In monkeys constant injection of small doses over a long period produced no symptoms; in guineapigs a subacute peritonitis, and in rabbits localised peritoneal growths.

The following details of these experiments are given in order to indicate the amount of work expended on this subject. Fifteen guineapigs were injected intra-peritoneally with 2 c.c. of a forty-eight hour broth culture of yeasts isolated from such various sources as thrush, air, sprue mouths, stools and post-mortems. On killing these animals some time after such a single injection no pathogenic lesions were found, nor could the organism be isolated from any of their tissues. The effect of prolonged injections was therefore tried, in weekly doses of a similar amount, but continued over a period of two months. The animals became ill and emaciated; post-mortem definite plastic peritonitis was found, but in only one case was I able to isolate yeasts from the tissues. In four rabbits single intraperitoneal injections produced no ill effects, but other results were obtained when the injections were constantly repeated. In one rabbit injected with a yeast isolated from a sprue liver definite tubercle-like lesions of the peritoneal surface of the liver and intestine were found post-mortem. A general infection with these yeasts had not, however, taken place and though in microscopical sections dead yeast cells were present in great numbers, yet cultures made direct from the growth proved to be sterile.

These experiments are of interest in view of the work of Roncali and Sanfelice on the *Saccharomyces neoformans* which they isolated from cancers and cancer-like growths and by injections of which they claimed to be able to reproduce similar tumours in experimental animals.

In my sections the structure of the tumour is that of a simple granuloma, though a few giant cells in which dead and encapsulated yeast cells can be demonstrated are found. Prolonged intraperitoneal injections with some other of my yeast cultures, such as a bakers' yeast, does not produce any such peritoneal growths.

Intraperitoneal injection of two monkeys with yeasts isolated from sprue tissues failed to produce any ill effects during life nor were any lesions found post-mortem.

Intravenous injections. The results of intravenous injections were of an entirely different character. Twenty-six separate experiments were made on rabbits, the injections, in doses of $\frac{1}{2}$–2 c.c., were made into the auricular veins with broth cultures obtained from different sources. Ten rabbits thus injected died in uraemic convulsions, generally from the third to twelfth day after injection. Post-mortem the kidneys were the only organs presenting any pathological changes; in these the cortex was, though not invariably, studded with minute yellow abscesses. Yeast cells could be recovered from the kidneys, spleen, liver and lungs in the majority of cases, but only in three instances from the heart's blood; the urine secreted by animals with definite kidney lesions was found to be swarming with yeasts.

All the yeasts in this series of experiments were isolated from sprue salivas, stools, or, post-mortem, from the intestines and organs of sprue cases. Control experiments were also made with cultures of the thrush organism *Monilia albicans* isolated from infants' mouths. The results obtained with one strain of this organism were similar to those I have just related, but another strain proved to be entirely harmless to rabbits even after repeated intravenous injection. On the other hand, variable results were obtained with my sprue yeasts when different animals and two separate cultures of the same organism were simultaneously employed, for although such an injection of a ½ c.c. of a sprue yeast culture proved fatal to one rabbit on one occasion, yet 8 c.c. of the same culture proved harmless to a second, nor could I recover the yeasts from the tissues after death.

Little could be learned from microscopical sections of the organs of these animals. In the cortex of the kidney numerous necrotic areas containing budding yeast cells and mycelial elements were present. The glomeruli appeared to be the starting point of the growth, though numbers of yeast cells could be found occasionally in the lumen of the convoluted tubules. In the walls of the vermiform appendix also, in one case, such a localised collection of cells was seen and yeasts were sparingly present in sections of the heart and spleen. Few changes as a rule, save fatty degeneration of a slight degree, were found in the liver, but in one instance round granular Gram-positive bodies were found in great abundance in the capillary endothelial cells resembling in their appearance and staining reactions the bodies found by me in the splenic veins of sprue.

Realising that the pathological changes just described were brought about by an overwhelming dose of the organism, I deemed it necessary to determine the effect in rabbits of repeated intravenous injections of minute doses of such pathogenic yeasts. Ten or more injections of the sprue yeasts, commencing with a dose of ½ c.c. gradually increased to 1 c.c. spaced out over a period of two months, were made on three rabbits. Two of these animals became intensely emaciated and anaemic and eventually died, while the third remained in good health. Post-mortem the kidneys showed no pathological changes; the organs, with one exception in which the last injection had been made but three days previous to death, were sterile on culture. On microscopical section giant cells, each enclosing one or more yeast cells, were found in the liver, whilst the organs of the other two were found to be normal. None of these experimental animals exhibited during life any symptoms suggestive of sprue, save perhaps the anaemia and intense emaciation, nor was any special wasting of the organs noted post-mortem.

I have so far only dealt with the pathogenic yeasts which I isolated from sprue post-mortems and stools, but I investigated twelve cultures obtained from other sources which were non-pathogenic to rabbits on intravenous injection. Such were yeasts isolated from the air[1],

---

[1] These organisms were apparently very numerous in the air in Ceylon; an average of twelve colonies from six 6 inch Petri dishes were cultivated on glucose-agar after an exposure of fifteen minutes in my laboratory.

rabbit and cow faeces, amoebic dysentery and normal stools, from bakers' yeast and from milk, and also from some sprue salivas and stools.

Constant intravenous injection with these non-pathogenic yeasts produced no ill effects on the animals employed nor any immunity to subsequent infection with those of the pathogenic series.

I also endeavoured to determine specific differences in these fungi by agglutination tests, but a short experience of the mode of growth of the yeast fungus in culture convinced me that the demonstration in this way of such an agglutination, if it does occur, was almost an impossibility. I therefore tried with crushed cultures of the organisms, but even by this means I failed to demonstrate any specific agglutination.

Evidence was not wanting, however, that after prolonged and continuous injection animals acquired a certain degree of tolerance to the pathogenic yeasts, and after several injections were not affected by double or even treble the preliminary dose.

I endeavoured also to ascertain whether the pathogenicity of these sprue yeasts and of *Monilia albicans* was directly due to the mechanical blockage of the renal capillaries by yeast cells or to some toxin excreted by them. I therefore injected two rabbits intravenously, on several occasions, with 10 c.c. of broth culture filtrate of such a pathogenic yeast. I failed to recognise any harmful effects that such injections may have had on these animals.

Although the results of these numerous experiments must be regarded as somewhat indefinite they seem to indicate that the sprue yeasts possess a certain degree of pathogenicity to rabbits on intravenous injection, a feature in which they agree with cultures of *Monilia albicans*, the thrush fungus, and that, though possessing the same morphological and cultural features, yet by these means they may be separated in the majority of yeasts from other sources.

(5) *The reactions with solutions of various sugars*

I attempted to classify the 106 yeast fungi isolated from many sources by means of their reactions with solutions of a limited number of sugars in the hope of finding a species peculiar to the sprue lesions.

On account of their rarity and cost I found it was impracticable to make use of all the fifteen sugars which Castellani employed for a similar purpose.

It was found that results of a practical nature were obtainable by using a 1 per cent. solution of six sugars in peptone water and by noting the reactions with litmus milk. The conclusion was reluctantly forced upon me that the results obtained from this line of research are quite untrustworthy as a guide to the classification of these organisms.

I will give my reasons very briefly for making what may seem to be a rather dogmatic statement.

Firstly, it was found that for the first ten days the longer the yeasts were cultured in their sugar solutions the more divergent were the ultimate reactions given by any particular culture (Appendix XIV A). I found, however, that after the tenth day in the incubator no further change in the fermentation reactions was produced. A provisional classification on the results of this ten days incubation was accordingly made (Appendix XIV B). It was found that my 106 cultures were divisible into fourteen types, but that all yeast cultures isolated from the same source and including the *Monilia albicans* derived from thrush were divisible into three or more species, and that in addition cultures recovered from the organs of an experimental rabbit gave completely different sugar reactions to those given by the organism with which the rabbit was originally injected intravenously (Appendix XIV B).

The conclusions made from these experiments received additional support by my subsequent work on the subject.

The sugar reactions of yeasts selected as examples of each provisional type were tested again at intervals of three months. For minute details of the results I must refer the reader to Appendix XIV C; suffice it to say that out of twelve types tested the reactions of only one remained constant on further subculture, and that any variation in the composition of the medium employed for dissolving the sugars, as for instance the substitution of broth for peptone water, had a very definite effect upon the ultimate reactions given by any particular yeast.

None of the organisms tested fermented mannite or affected litmus milk in any way.

As a result of this rather tedious work I felt justified in abandoning the classification of these organisms on a basis which has been so extensively employed by Castellani in his differentiation of species, and in concluding that no specific distinction between the *Monilia albicans* and the yeast organism found in sprue tissues could be substantiated.

I have summed up in the next Chapter the evidence I have collected in favour of and the evidence against the thrush fungus *Monilia albicans* being the primary cause of sprue.

CHAPTER XVII

*Evidence in favour of and against regarding sprue as a
blastomycotic infection*

(1) YEAST cells and mycelial elements are found situated intracellularly in scrapings of the tongue lesions at an early stage of the
disease and cannot be found in scrapings made from the former site
of the lesion at a later stage when symptoms have subsided.

(2) Yeasts are the only organisms found in the deeper layers of
the tongue in microscopical sections. The evidence that the infection
is not of recent date receives support from the chronic inflammatory
changes in the epidermis and the corium of the papillae and from
the presence of Russell's bodies in this situation.

(3) The desquamation of the epithelial cells accompanied by a
subacute inflammation of the tongue and of the oesophagus are changes
such as would be expected from a study of the mode of growth of the
fungus and of its low order of virulence.

(4) A general infection of the intestinal mucus with yeasts was
found in sprue post-mortems but no such general infection was found
in other chronic wasting diarrhoeas.

(5) The stools of sprue, their frothy and gaseous character, are
such as one would expect in a blastomycotic infection of the intestinal
canal.

(6) The relapsing nature, the chronicity and latency of the disease
are symptoms such as one would expect from a knowledge of the life
history of the blastomyces, their periods of attenuated growth and of
sudden recrudescences.

(7) There is no evidence in favour of regarding the sprue yeast
fungus as being otherwise than identical with the thrush fungus,
Monilia albicans, an organism possessing a very low pathogenic power,
but it is possible that under certain unknown conditions, more or less

peculiar to the tropics, this power may become greatly augmented. In support of this view I may add that it is a well recognised fact that there are endless varieties of yeasts employed in the brewing of beer and in making wine, and that the predominance of a variety in certain districts imparts to the local wine its characteristic flavour, and which, though differing widely from each other in their powers of growth and fermentation, yet resemble each other minutely in their morphological and cultural characters. May it not be that the pathogenic yeasts can be similarly altered by local conditions! I surmise that under certain circumstances these fungi, though normally non-pathogenic, are capable of assuming a pathogenic *rôle*, as is known to happen in the case of the *pneumococcus*, the diphtheria bacillus, the *Micrococcus catarrhalis*, and probably in the case of the *Entamoeba histolytica* as well.

That the thrush fungus is capable of causing a desquamation of the epidermis of the lingual papillae there can be little doubt; in sections stained by Giemsa the epithelial cells in the immediate vicinity are vacuolated and in some places completely destroyed, thus laying bare the subjacent connective tissue; there is an intense inflammatory change in the immediate vicinity; the nuclei of the epithelial cells have undergone chromatolysis; the epithelial layer itself is crowded with polymorphonuclear cells, not usually found in this situation; the capillaries of the corium are dilated and filled with leucoytes,—all evidences of a reaction on the part of the tissues invaded by the fungus. (Plate IV, fig. 3.) Of one thing there can be little doubt, namely that this injection is not the result of a post-mortem ingrowth.

Exactly the same changes are visible in the oesophagus where there are also collections of inflammatory cells in the subjacent mucous and aveolar coats.

There can be little doubt, as a result of my studies, that these fungi in their downward growth are capable of exposing the taste buds and nerve terminals and of causing the very lesions, which the lingual and oesophageal symptoms of sprue suggest are present.

(8) Wasting and anaemia, both symptoms of sprue, can be produced in rabbits by continuous intravenous injections of small doses of a broth culture of such a pathogenic yeast; moreover a degeneration of the capillary endothelial cells of the liver, apparently similar to the degeneration found in the sprue spleen, may be produced in these animals by the same means.

(9) Diarrhoea, atrophy of the lingual papillae (as in sprue), digestive disturbances and aphthous ulceration of the mouth are commonly found in infants, the subjects of a thrush infection in temperate zones.

(10)   It is possible that obscure alimentary diseases of children in temperate zones, such as Gee's coeliac diarrhoea[1], are of the same nature as sprue in adults in the tropics.   A hypothesis of this sort would explain the occurrence of sporadic cases of sprue in temperate zones.

(11)   The local affection of different portions of the digestive tract with this fungus would best explain the varying clinical manifestations of sprue.

(12)   To maintain such a hypothesis, it is necessary to stipulate for a third factor, a predisposing cause, which may exist in local tropical climatic conditions, conditions which favour a more precocious and luxuriant growth of all the fungi, a matter of common observation to all laboratory workers in the tropics.

Evidence against regarding sprue as a blastomycotic infection

(1)   Thrush (*Monilia albicans*) is a terminal, though uncommon, infection in other chronic wasting diseases such as phthisis, cancer, diabetes, etc.

(2)   General infections of the alimentary canal with this fungus have been reported in temperate zones.

(3)   If the geographical distribution of sprue be eventually found to correspond with that of other typically tropical diseases, such a fact alone is in favour of a protozoal rather than a fungoid or bacterial origin of the disease.

---

[1] Gee's coeliac diarrhoea, first described in 1868, is a chronic wasting disorder of childhood, characterised by diarrhoea, by large, pale, fermenting and offensive stools, running a prolonged course with tendency to relapse, which may end in death or in complete recovery, or in partial recovery with consequent impairment of growth and of development.   The disease generally commences in the second or third year of life, and is accompanied by anaemia, oedema of the extremities, great emaciation and abdominal distension. Little is known about the pathology; there is said to be an atrophy of the intestinal canal.   Several theories have been advanced implicating the activity of organs such as the liver and the pancreas.

CHAPTER XVIII

TREATMENT

My limited experience of sprue does not permit me to attempt an extended discussion of the whole subject of treatment. I will here record only my own experiences, and with special reference to Ceylon.

I was able to observe the results of treatment in seven cases of typical sprue and five cases of chronic diarrhoea who were under my immediate personal care in Nuwara Eliya, but in addition to this number I was able to watch the effects of similar treatment in numerous other cases scattered over the island.

My results were with one exception (case 6) encouraging, but at this early date it is impossible to say whether the manifest improvement has been maintained or that relapses will occur in the future. The methods I employed did not differ from those laid down and practised with so much success by Thin, Manson and others, save that I had the advantage of a stock of fresh bael fruit which I used in every case and which I concluded is of a distinct medicinal value in the treatment of the disease.

With the exception of bael fruit, which I employed in an entirely empirical manner, I regulated the dietary by the patients' symptoms, such as the condition of mouth, the dyspepsia, the number, colour and size of the stools, taking any increase or decrease in body weight as a rough guide.

The favourable results I obtained I am inclined to ascribe partly to the cool climate of Nuwara Eliya where the cases were treated, and partly to the supply of fresh milk from *English* cows, so essential but generally unobtainable in the hot plains. I wish to lay special stress on the removal of sprue patients from the heat into a cooler and more equitable climate, as I am aware that there exists a prejudice in Ceylon against removal to a high altitude. It is said that an uncontrollable diarrhoea will ensue on such removal. My experience is diametrically opposed to this. In no patient, when every precaution was taken to guard against chill, was the removal from the low-country to Nuwara Eliya followed by diarrhoea. I am inclined to regard this change of climate as the most important factor in the treatment of the disease, and I am able to cite one case (case 5) in support of this statement. Here was an acute case treated in Colombo on identically the same lines as I subsequently adopted in Nuwara Eliya, but who had made no progress there. His improvement directly he was removed to Nuwara Eliya was manifest and remarkable; all symptoms rapidly disappeared and he put on a total of 34 lbs. body weight in the comparatively short period of thirty-seven days.

Though this was an exceptional instance, · the improvement in my other patients, one of whom it should be noted was over seventy years of age, encourages me to believe that the treatment of the disease can be as efficiently carried out in the hill stations of Ceylon, as it can be in Europe. The practice adopted by many medical men in the tropics, of banishing the victim of sprue from the endemic area directly signs of the disease appear, is, I believe, much to be deprecated in many instances. I am sure the chances of eventual recovery are in a proportion of cases jeopardised by this practice. Such patients are often acutely ill. All their symptoms are apt to be aggravated by the sea journey; the dyspepsia by the motion of the ship and possibly by sea-sickness; the diarrhoea by the unsuitable food; fresh milk is unobtainable and the frozen and preserved substitutes provided by Eastern steamship companies are unpalatable and often quite unsuitable for sprue patients. Is it to be wondered at that under these conditions quite a number of sprue cases die at sea? On the other hand should it be deemed advantageous for the patient to return to Europe, I submit that my experience of the treatment of the disease in Ceylon renders a preliminary course, such as I adopted in Nuwara Eliya, advisable, if not essential.

In order to make my statements on this subject more explicit I subjoin a short account of the treatment and its results in Nuwara Eliya of seven cases of typical sprue and five cases of chronic diarrhoea of probably the same nature.

Details of cases

Cases of typical sprue

(1)   Planter, male, aet 56, ill two years; tall spare man, large stools, subacute mouth and marked dyspeptic symptoms. Great improvement under treatment for forty-two days in Nuwara Eliya, increase of 22½ lbs. in weight from 10 st. 7 lbs. to 12 st. 1½ lbs. Methods employed: diet milk and bael fruit, pot. chlorate mouth wash after food, pepâna tabloids after meals, iron and arsenic injections. Diet increased from milk, 3 pints to 5, bananas, toast, jellies and puddings, eventually shredded meat added. Blood, increase in red cells from 2,000,000 to 4,037,000, haemoglobin from 70–100 per cent. Weight remained the same for a year then had a relapse.

(2)   Planter, male, aet 45, ill six months, tongue symptoms subacute, diarrhoea acute, slight febrile temperature, dyspepsia marked; emaciation extreme, large pale stools. Improvement under treatment for forty-three days in Nuwara Eliya, increase of 25 lbs. in weight—from 7 st. 2½ lbs. to 9 stone. Methods employed: milk 3 pints gradually increased to 5 pints, bael fruit, jellies, pot. chlorate mouth wash, small doses of castor oil, iron and arsenic injections. Relapse due to chill and mental symptoms. Returned to estate where he has since lived on a light diet and fruit and has remained free from symptoms. Blood, increase of red cells from 2,700,000 to 4,000,000; haemoglobin from 65–100 per cent.

(3)   Merchant, male, aet 41, ill two years; diarrhoea acute and cyclical, no tongue symptoms. At first loss of weight (from 8 st. 13 lbs. to 8 st. 4 lbs.); treated in Nuwara Eliya for forty-four days. Great improvement in well-being, diarrhoea ceased. Methods employed: rest in bed, milk diet, gruel, bananas, chicken broth, bael fruit, castor oil in small doses, pepâna tabloids. Returned to work in Colombo, subsequent increase in weight to 9 stone, has remained well ever since and now weighs 10 st. 4 lbs. (Feb. 1914).

(4)   Planter, male, aet 70, ill three years; diarrhoea acute (nine stools a day), tongue symptoms marked, treated in Nuwara Eliya hospital for forty-three days. Emetine injections given for diarrhoea, but with no effect. Milk and bael fruit disagreed. Great improvement on steamed and shredded beef. Severe set back owing to constipation and faecal impaction, eventually great improvement. Left hospital weighing 9 st., returned to England where he has continued to put on weight and now weighs 10 st. 12 lbs. and is eating full diet, no further symptoms up to date.

(5)   Burgher, male, aet 23, ill six months; treated in Colombo General Hospital, but steadily getting thinner and diarrhoea worse; diarrhoea and mouth symptoms severe, great improvement under treatment in Nuwara Eliya for fifty-three days, increase in weight of 34 lbs. in thirty-seven days from 8 st. 7 lbs. to 10 st. 13 lbs. Methods employed: milk diet 3 pints, bael fruit, diet gradually increased, stools become smaller and darker; small doses of castor oil, intra-muscular injections of iron and arsenic. Left to take up appointment in Malay States in good health. Blood, increase of red cells from 2,000,000 to 5,000,000; haemoglobin from 70–100 per cent.

(6)   Female, aet 36, seen first in Colombo; ill one year; mouth symptoms and diarrhoea acute. Treated in Nuwara Eliya Hospital for twenty-seven days.

Methods employed: milk, bael fruit, castor oil; patient refused to carry out treatment, so was discharged, subsequently relapsed, passed from one hospital to another and eventually died in Colombo General Hospital.—Autopsy post-mortem A.

(7) Planter's wife, aet 43, ill for three years. Treated for sprue in England in 1911, subsequently in Bath on santonin. In July 1912 had a relapse. Tongue symptoms and diarrhoea marked. Treated in bungalow on tea estate. Rest in bed, milk, bael fruit, castor oil, rapidly put on weight, 5 lbs. in three weeks, alkaline mouth wash, injections of iron and arsenic. Has remained well.

(For further details of diet, medicinal treatment, weight of stools, etc. of these cases, the reader is referred to Appendix XV.)

Cases of chronic diarrhoea (probably early cases of sprue)

(8) Planter, male, aet 33, ill two years with diarrhoea, no tongue symptoms, frothy bilious early morning stools; no amoebae, but many yeast cells. Returned subsequently to England and on a light diet recovered, remained well and returned to Ceylon.

(9) Planter, male, aet 25, ill six months, no tongue symptoms, frothy bilious early morning stools, no amoebae found. Treatment in bed, one week, milk and bael fruit, good recovery.

(10) Planter, male, aet 22, ill four months, no tongue symptoms, bilious frothy early morning stools, no amoebae found; completely recovered on diet and subsequently returned to England.

(11) Planter, male, aet 27, ill three months, no tongue symptoms, bilious frothy early morning stools, no amoebae found. Treatment in bed, milk and bael fruit,—relapsed—treated again on same lines and recovered. Has remained well.

(12) Planter, male, aet 20. Ill five weeks, diarrhoea, no tongue symptoms, bilious frothy early morning stools, no amoebae found. Progressive emaciation, feeling of lassitude, distension of abdomen, aphthae in mouth. Treatment: rest in bed fourteen days, milk, bael fruit, jellies, rapid improvement, eventual recovery.

I propose to discuss shortly the various methods of treatment I employed under the head of (a) general, (b) dietetic, and (c) medicinal measures.

(a) General measures

The avoidance of chill is a matter that does not require to be emphasised. I advised my patients on their journey to Nuwara Eliya to wear the warmest clothes procurable; on arrival the patients were immediately placed in bed and a fire was kept up in the sick room especially at night time. I insisted on complete mental and bodily rest for a period of three weeks, after which the patients were allowed a gradual increasing amount of exercise. Twice I learned, through temporary recrudescence of the mouth symptoms and the diarrhoea, how carefully such out-door exercise needs to be regulated.

The strain entailed in walking an extra half-mile or the exposure to a short rain-storm were quite sufficient to undo all the good derived from the treatment of the previous month.

(b) *Dietetic measures*

Milk. The best milk from English cows procurable was given. I learned the importance of testing the milk frequently and to regard with suspicion any sample of a specific gravity below 1030 as being adulterated with water of doubtful purity, a favourite practice of the native milk vendors.

On account of the uncertainty of its source, even in Nuwara Eliya, it is the usual practice with Europeans in Ceylon to boil all milk. For the treatment of sprue I found it inadvisable to do so for several reasons. Boiling renders milk not only more unpalatable, but less easily digestible, than plain; I found the best results were obtained by heating it to 140° F. for twenty minutes before use; the patient was then advised to sip the milk slowly after it had cooled down to body temperature. I generally commenced treatment with about three pints and gradually increased the amount by a daily addition of half a pint till five and a half pints were reached, which amount I found was about the maximum quantity a patient could digest or tolerate in the twenty-four hours. Eight ounce feeds were given two-hourly during the daytime and three times during the night. As the treatment proceeded, the practice I adopted was gradually to increase the amount and to reduce the number of meals in the twenty-four hours.

Meat. Two patients could not well tolerate or digest the milk diet; I decided to substitute for milk small quantities of underdone and shredded steamed beef. There is considerable difficulty in procuring meat of requisite nutritive quality and tenderness in Nuwara Eliya. I selected the most tender steak undercut procurable and minced it very fine, subsequently steaming the mince for ten minutes in a porcelain vessel suspended in boiling water. As a substitute for one of the morning milk feeds I commenced with four ounces of this mince, to which, to render it more palatable, a little pepper and salt had been added. Subsequently I increased the amount of meat and decreased the amount of milk. Under this treatment the patient's symptoms rapidly ameliorated and the hitherto uncontrolled diarrhoea ceased.

Fruit. Many fruits were tried. The most suitable and most easily procurable locally was the banana, which was usually given as a sort of purée mashed up with cream and sugar. I allowed my convalescent cases to consume sixteen or more bananas a day without untoward results. Care must be taken to distinguish between the banana and the variety known as the plantain, the latter, a coarse and unpalatable fruit containing five cells on cross-section to three of the banana, is sold by the natives in the up-country districts and is quite unsuitable for sprue patients.

The peculiar flavour of the pawpaw (*Carica papaya*), which can be procured in all seasons in Ceylon, is not agreeable to every one; the pulp, however, is easily digestible and contains a digestive ferment *papaine* which may be of distinct benefit, especially in cases in which gastric symptoms predominate. The Avocado pear (*Pusea gratissima*) was occasionally tried; it is a greasy and fatty fruit, and its use was not followed by favourable results.

Australian grapes and apples were also given a trial. Grapes are very acceptable and do not appear to aggravate the mouth symptoms; on the other hand I was inclined to doubt the advisability of giving apples, either raw or baked, during convalescence.

Diet during convalescence. During convalescence I found that quantities and varieties of other articles of diet could be gradually introduced, beginning with jellies, such as plain calves foot and fruit jellies, overcooked rice and milk puddings, pounded "seer fish" in very small quantities, and soups, such as Bovril and chicken broth. I advised my patients to live on white meat, such as chicken, as long as they were able and to postpone a return to "estate beef" as long as possible. The method proposed by Manson to convalescents, of adopting a daily Sunday fast of milk combined with mild purgation, I found to be a very useful one.

(c) *Medicinal measures*

These were few and simple. Small doses of castor oil ($\mathfrak{z}$ss.—$\mathfrak{z}$i) in gelatin capsules, as sold by Parke, Davis and Co., were given every night, *whether the diarrhoea continued or not.* Such a course ensures a daily and painless evacuation and is calculated to clear away any excess of mucus clinging to the secretory surface of the bowel. The patients with mouth symptoms were advised to cleanse the mouth with a mild alkaline potassium chlorate mouth wash (grs. x to the ounce of water) after every meal; this I consider a most important measure and one which is often neglected.

I found the application of a silver nitrate stick speedily caused the disappearance of the aphthae; for sore patches on the tongue the application of a solution of borax in glycerin was of distinct value. For the dyspeptic symptoms a mixture of bismuth and soda was used sometimes with advantage, but as a general rule more benefit accrued from pancreatic preparations. The pepâna tabloids, as prepared by Burroughs and Wellcome, given after every meal gave the best results. Taka-diastase preparations of Parke, Davis and Co., were also of distinct advantage in some cases, while Savory and Moore's pancreatic emulsion—in doses of two teaspoonsfull in a teacup of milk one hour after meals—seemed rather to aggravate the symptoms in the only case I tried it.

Six or more intramuscular injections of iron and arsenic as prepared by Molteni, or similar preparations by Burroughs and Wellcome, were given at intervals of three days during the convalescent period and appeared not only to improve the condition of the blood but also the patient's general well-being.

The one medicinal measure which experience taught me to estimate as being of distinct value was the bael fruit (*Aegle marmelos*) the use of which was first brought to the notice of European practitioners by Fayrer ((1878), *Med. Times and Gaz.* 611 and 645). It is a large globose fruit with a hard wooden rind and contains an astringent yellow pulp with a peculiar flavour, reminiscent of an over-ripe peach. The pulp is composed of ten to sixteen cells each lodging an oval seed embedded in a viscid and transparent mucus with a terebinthinate flavour. The medicinal properties appear to reside in tannic acid, in an essential oil and in a bitter principle. In England it is obtainable as the dried fruit or as the liquid extract, neither of which forms appear to possess the medicinal properties of the fresh ripe fruit, though latterly a bottled preparation is exported from India and sold by the Army and Navy Stores in which the properties of the fresh fruit may be expected to be preserved in a more efficient state than in the old and dried preparations.

In Ceylon bael fruit is generally obtainable at all seasons. Though it is not specially cultivated, it grows everywhere in abundance in the low-country and up to an elevation of 1800 feet. It occurs in a small and large variety and ripens at two distinct seasons of the year according as it is grown in Colombo or in Kandy.

I found it advisable to give one large or two small fruits during the day. If given in an unripe state or in too large amount it seems to cause dyspepsia. In its most favourable condition the pulp has all the characteristics already referred to, but, if kept an undue length of time before use, it rapidly becomes overgrown with moulds.

There are various methods of administering the fruit which it is advisable to refer to briefly. It is best given in a raw state; the soft pulp scraped out of the shell by a fork, thus leaving only the fibrous matrix behind, should be well mixed with sugar and cream and partaken of in small amounts with each feed of milk. To some people the raw fruit is unpalatable, and to these it may be given in the form of bael fruit tea. For this purpose a whole fruit is split open, toasted in front of the fire, infused with hot water, mixed with sugar and milk and sipped like tea. Or an extract of the pulp may be mashed up into the consistency of a "gooseberry fool," strained through muslin, mixed with gelatin and made into a jelly, the flavour of which is much improved by the addition of a wineglassful of sherry.

The resinous substances contained in the fruit are apparently excreted unchanged in the stools and when mixed with strong sulphuric acid a blood-red reaction results; a reaction which is also given by the undigested pulp. I was unable to ascertain whether any of the active principles of the fruit were excreted in the urine, which certainly acquires during the use of the fruit a peculiar and somewhat cat-like smell; but does not give the reaction just referred to.

I advised bael fruit to certain sprue cases, whom I was unable to treat for any length of time and I had uniformly good reports of its effects.

Santonin. I interviewed seven cases of sprue who had been treated with yellow santonin as advised and so ardently advocated by Begg. Of the total number I only found one who considered it was of value. Since his return to the island this patient has been in the habit of using the drug when suffering from recrudescences of the disease. I was unable to convince myself that santonin treatment is of any specific value in sprue.

"*Batavia powder*," or powdered cuttle-fish bone, "Mrs Brown's Singapore cure," or powdered mangosteen rinds, "Rhein's specific," or powdered cuttle-fish bone and crabs' eyes, were all procured and enquired into. I could obtain no evidence that they were of any special value in actually curing the disease, though they may be of use in checking intercurrent attacks of diarrhoea.

Appendicectomy is a heroic measure which appears to be of little value. I saw three cases on whom this operation had been performed and whose condition seemed to be rather aggravated than ameliorated thereby.

Emetine injections up to gr. i per diem were tried in three cases with violent diarrhoea; as might be expected it was found to be of no value.

The treatment of complications

The most frequent complication of sprue, if such it can be called, was constipation. For this I was in the habit of giving gradually increased doses of castor oil, and if this failed, a soap and water enema.

One case (case 4) previously operated on for haemorrhoids with consequent stenosis of the anal orifice suffered acutely for several days from faecal impaction which eventually necessitated the removal of hard faecal lumps from the rectum by means of a spoon and the daily injection of soap and water enemata. Subsequently the bowels were satisfactorily regulated by medicinal paraffin given in drachm doses every night.

Undue worry, culminating in insomnia and mental symptoms, caused a severe set back in one of my cases, but removal of the patient from hospital to his estate amidst familiar surroundings rapidly banished these symptoms and was followed by an immediate improvement in his physical and mental condition. This patient had a slight fever also—up to 100° F.—every night; there was no other local cause to account for the rise of temperature. From the fact that it became normal during convalescence directly the diarrhoea had ceased, I inferred that it was due to the absorption of some toxic matter from the bowel wall.

After treatment. In estimating the value of any medicinal treatment one must not lose sight of the fact that many cases of sprue occurring in Ceylon have recovered with no other treatment than their own common sense suggested. From the details of some of these cases I must refer the reader to Appendix XVI where under cases 8 and 11 he will find the record of gentlemen now in perfect health who in the past had undoubtedly suffered from sprue and who, being able to leave the colony, had treated themselves with bismuth and castor oil, and had completely recovered and had since remained in good health.

Return to the endemic area after a cure in Europe

Return to the endemic area after an apparent recovery from sprue is contrary to the advice generally given by most authorities. Whether this is sound advice or not is problematical. I must refer the reader once more to the twelve cases recorded in Appendix XVI for my reasons for making this statement; there he will find instances of residents who, since their return from a cure in England, have remained in perfect health for a period of twenty years. There are also two remarkable cases (cases 6 and 9) both of whom lost nearly half their total body weight during their illness and who, ever since their return to the endemic area where they contracted the disease, have continued steadily to improve until they have fully regained their normal body weight. In case 6 there are other points to be noted. It will be seen that this gentleman suffered from a severe recrudescence of symptoms directly he landed in the Colony and that, contrary to medical advice, he returned to his estate in Galle, a very hot and damp locality, and without any medical aid whatsoever, even while pursuing his daily avocations, he continued to improve on a diet of milk, eggs and fruit, to such an extent that when I saw him in December 1912, that is a year after his return to the colony, he was in perfect health.

After a consideration of these cases and of others whom I treated in the Colony, with whom I have kept in touch ever since, I am not inclined to regard sprue, unless it has proceeded to a high degree of destruction of the glandular and absorbent structures of the alimentary canal, as being invariably either a fatal or an incurable disease. If so how account for these genuine and remarkable recoveries?

CHAPTER XIX

DIFFERENTIAL DIAGNOSIS

I HAVE already alluded to the difficulty of diagnosing sprue in natives; in Europeans, on the other hand, many of these difficulties do not present themselves and therefore one has but to differentiate the sprue diarrhoea from others of undoubted specific origin.

Diarrhoeas in Europeans

Of these a diarrhoea associated with and consequent upon amoebic dysentery is by far the most important and though in many cases I was able satisfactorily to demonstrate the *Entamoeba histolytica* and its nucleated cysts in the stools, yet there were others in which the therapeutic tests only—the administration of emetine—made such a differentiation possible. I therefore came to regard emetine as the sole reliable means of differentiating diarrhoea of dysenteric origin from other forms of intestinal flux. I treated nine cases, mostly young planters and their wives, who though giving a past history of traces of blood and mucus in their stools, had been suffering—in one case for six years—from a violent explosive early morning diarrhoea, without any involvement of the tongue. On examining the stools microscopically I discovered, in four cases only, a few vegetative amoebae and cysts with four nuclei sparingly distributed in the faecal matter. In only one case was there any appreciable amount of mucus present in the stool. The nature of the other five cases could only be inferred by the specific and miraculous action of emetine upon them. In only two of the series could any thickening of the sigmoid flexure of the colon be made out by an abdominal examination. I do not propose to burden the text with details of these cases of which I have kept full records. Suffice it to say that emetine hydrochloride was injected hypodermically in doses of $\frac{2}{3}$ gr. daily for the first few days of treatment, subsequently for a week in doses of $\frac{1}{3}$ grain every night. While under this treatment I allowed a certain amount of exercise, such as curtailed rounds of golf. All these cases made an excellent recovery and did not subsequently suffer from a relapse. One case had previously been operated upon for a liver abscess and two had undergone appendicectomy. It is probable that the inflammation of the appendix in the two latter instances was of amoebic origin and could have been appropriately treated by other means than by operation. Were the frequency of amoebic ulceration of the vermiform appendix borne in mind by tropical physicians, the hypodermic injection of emetine would be found safer and more efficient in many cases than the surgeon's knife.

By the same means I treated successfully three obvious cases of amoebic dysentery; also a gentleman who suffered from recurrent febrile attacks, probably consequent on a subacute hepatitis, but in whom, however, no hepatic enlargement could be elicited by physical examination. Two of the cases subsequently relapsed, but recovered eventually on resuming the same treatment. I found it was advisable, after a preliminary course of emetine treatment, such as outlined above, to continue the injections in doses of one-third of a grain with alternate intervals of a week's rest for a month or longer. The ultimate result of this method was to prevent any further relapse.

The hypodermic injection was followed in a few instances by a subacute inflammation of the surrounding skin, but beyond this no untoward symptoms whatsoever ensued.

Diarrhoeas in natives

Diarrhoeas of amoebic origin are of frequent occurrence amongst the plantation coolies and undoubtedly account for a number of the deaths at present included under the heading "Diarrhoea." The existence of this amoebic diarrhoea is not sufficiently recognised by medical officers in charge of estates. Were these coolies efficiently treated with emetine, either hypodermically or orally in keratin capsules, before the condition is beyond hope of recovery, I am sure that the mortality from "Diarrhoea," now such a serious obstacle to progress and such a financial loss to estates, would be soon much reduced.

Diarrhoea as a terminal symptom of ankylostomiasis

I performed twelve post-mortems on Tamil and Sinhalese coolies in whom diarrhoea had been the most prominent symptom in life, and in whom the numerous ankylostomes found in the small intestine constituted the only ascertainable cause of their fatal illnesses.

In no instance had the presence of ankylostomiasis been diagnosed during life, or the appropriate treatment applied, even though many other such obvious signs of the disease, as oedema and anaemia, were present. During life the diarrhoea was intense and the motions were light coloured and sometimes frothy; the tongue was naturally pale and anaemic, but the papillae were not atrophied. The tissues were examined microscopically in all these cases, but no invasion of the tongue or oesophagus by the thrush organism was seen, though in the sections of the gut some round cell infiltration could be made out.

One is justified in regarding the ankylostome in these cases as being a primary infection and the diarrhoea as a terminal phenomenon, or perhaps as a secondary infection of the intestine by some micro-organism. It is not improbable that a microscopical examination of the stools for ova and the application of the appropriate antihelminthic treatment in these cases would not only have checked the diarrhoea, but also have saved the patients. Were the existence of this ankylostome diarrhoea more generally recognised by district medical officers, the formidable number of deaths now registered under the heading of "Diarrhoea" would be reduced.

CHAPTER XX

CONCLUSIONS

1. Sprue is a specific disease of tropical and subtropical countries, though it is possible that cases occasionally originate in temperate zones.

2. It is a prevalent disease in Ceylon, especially amongst the Europeans. Contrary to the opinion hitherto held, it occurs amongst the natives irrespective of race or mode of life.

3. This fact, together with the occurrence of the disease in people closely associated with one another, suggests some specific local influence or some communication of the specific cause from man to man.

4. Sprue is a variable disease. It may occur in a mild or in a particularly virulent form, and, in common with many other serious diseases, is prone to sudden exacerbations, remissions and periods of latency.

5. There is evidence that the disease may occur as distinct clinical forms according to the portion of the alimentary canal attacked.

6. Researches on the composition of the stools point either to a complete absence or to inadequacy of the intestinal digestive ferments.

7. Researches on the blood and on the urine are in favour of regarding certain of the more important clinical features of sprue as dependent on an alimentary toxaemia.

8. **The pathological findings are also in favour of such a conclusion and, if anything, point to an infection with the thrush fungus (*Monilia albicans*) as being the cause**[1].

[1] I realise that I have been unable to demonstrate in microscopical sections any invasion of the intestinal mucosa by yeast fungi in the same manner as takes place in the oesophagus and in the tongue, but having found an overgrowth of these organisms in the mucus lining the intestinal canal, I was led to stipulate for the excretion and absorption of some irritative toxin from this layer of mucus capable of giving rise to the chronic inflammatory changes in the mucosa and capable of prohibiting, or in some way nullifying, the action of the intestinal and pancreatic ferments. I therefore instituted some experiments designed to ascertain whether the presence of these yeast fungi, or an extract of such a culture, were capable of neutralising the ferments in an artificial pancreatic preparation.

For this purpose a culture of the fungus was placed in an Erlenmeyer flask and an equal quantity of Benger's "Liquor Pancreaticus" 1·30 dissolved in 1 per cent. sodium bicarbonate, was added. 2 grammes of Merck's prepared fibrin suspended in a muslin bag was immersed in this mixture and incubated for a period of twenty-four hours at 37° C.

As compared with control preparations I was quite unable to demonstrate any such inhibitive action.

It is possible to account for the apparent absence of the pancreatic juice in other ways. It may be that the mucosa of the duodenum and jejunum are affected to such a degree as to prevent the formation of *secretin* and its consequent stimulating action of the pancreas (Bayliss and Starling), or again it is possible that the conversion of *trypsinogen* to *trypsin* has been prevented by the insufficiency or complete lack of the *succus entericus*.

CHAPTER XXI

BIBLIOGRAPHY

English References to Sprue

ALLBUTT and ROLLESTON (1907). *System of Medicine.* 2nd edit. II. pt. 2, 545.

ANNESLEY (1831). *Sketches of the most Prevalent Diseases of India.* London.

—— (1841). *Researches into the Diseases of India.* London.

ASHFORD, B. K. (viii. 1913). Notes on Sprue in Porto Rico and the results of Treatment by Santonin. *Am. Journ. Trop. Dis. and Prev. Med.* I. 146–158.

BALY (1847). Goultstonian Lectures. *Lond. Med. Gaz.* XXXIX. 441.

BASSETT-SMITH, P. W. (1903). Discussion on Sprue. *Brit. Med. Journ.* II. 641–644.

BEGG, CHAS. (1887). Psilosis or Sprue or Diarrhoea. *China Imp. Marit. Customs Med. Rep.* 34th issue, 32.

—— (1898). Santonin in Sprue. *Lancet,* I. 185, 244.

—— (1907). Complications found in chronic cases of Sprue. *Journ. Trop. Med.* X. 293.

—— (1912). Sprue, its Diagnosis and Treatment.

BLACK, J. R. (1888). Two Cases of Sprue. *Glas. Med. Journ.* XXIX. 473.

BRUNTON, LAUDER (1900). Sprue. *Edin. Med. Journ.* N.S. VII. 105–113.

BUCHANAN and others (1899). A Discussion on Psilosis or Sprue. *Journ. Trop. Med.* II. 43–49.

BURG, VAN DER (1883–4). *China Imp. Marit. Customs Med. Rep.* 27th issue, 55.

CAMMIDGE (1905). Observations on the Faeces in Biliary Obstruction and Pancreatic Disease. *Brit. Med. Journ.* II. 1102–1104.

—— (1907). Complications found in chronic cases of Sprue. *Journ. Trop. Med.* X. 293.

CANTLIE, CLARK, and others (1903). Discussion on Sprue. *Brit. Med. Journ.* II. 644.

CANTLIE (1906). Sprue and Intestinal Lesions. *Journ. Trop. Med.* IX. 277–279.

—— (1907). Ipecacuanha in Sprue. *Idem.* X. 294.

—— (1913). Collosol argentum. Its use in Sprue and Post-dysenteric conditions. *Journ. Trop. Med.* 123, 124; also *Brit. Med. Journ.* II. 1296, 1297.

CARNEGIE-BROWN (1908). Sprue and its Treatment.

CASTELLANI, A. (1912). Note on Certain Cell Inclusions. *Journ. Trop. Med.* XV. 354.

CASTELLANI and CHALMERS (1913). *Manual of Tropical Medicine.* 2nd edit. 1325.

CASTELLANI, A. and Low, G. C. (1913). The Role played by fungi in Sprue. *Journ. Trop. Med.* XVI. 34.

COUPLAND (1881). Sprue [Editorial]. *Brit. Med. Journ.* I. 524.

CROMBIE (1880). Particulars regarding the prevalence of diarrhoea at Simla in 1880. *Ind. Med. Gaz.* XV. 313.

CUNNINGHAM (1877). *14th Ann. Rep. of the San. Commiss. of the Govt. of India,* 123.

DANIELS, C. W. (1912). *Trop. Med. and Hygiene*, pt. III.

DONALD, W. D. (1881). Sprue—Ceylon sore Mouth. *Brit. Med. Journ.* I. 661.

FAYRER, J. (1878). On the Bael Fruit, etc. *Med. Times and Gaz.* I. 611, 645.

—— (1878). The Bael Fruit. *Ibid.* II. 86.

—— (1881). *Tropical Dysentery and Chronic Diarrhoea.* London, 127.

—— (1893). Tropical Diarrhoea. Davidson's *Hygiene and Diseases of Warm Climates*, 521.

GALLOWAY, D. J. (1905). Some Clinical Notes on the Etiology of Sprue. *Journ. Trop. Med.* VIII. 289.

—— (1905). The Treatment of Sprue. *Ibid.* VIII. 301–304.

GRAHAM, J. C. (1905). Discussion on Sprue and Hill Diarrhoea. *Brit. Med. Journ.* II. 1284.

HARLEY and GOODBODY (1906). *Chemical Investigations of the Gastric and Intestinal Diseases.*

HARTIGAN, N. (1905). The Use of Cyllin in Sprue. *Journ. Trop. Med.* VIII. 65.

HILLARY (1766). *Observations on the Changes of Air and the Concomitant Epidemical Diseases in the Island of Barbados.* London. 2nd edit.

HORTON (1874). *The Diseases of Tropical Climates.* London.

HUNTER, F. S. (1909). Notes on Tropical Diarrhoea. *Trans. Bombay Med. Congress.*

JEFFERYS and MAXWELL (1910). *Diseases of China.* London, 228–230.

LOW, G. C. (1912). The Blood in Sprue. *Journ. Trop. Med.* XV. 130.

—— (1914). Arthritis in Sprue. *Ibid.* XVII. 1.

MACLEAN (1886). *Lectures on the Diseases of Tropical Countries.* London.

MACY, F. S. (1909). Notes on Tropical Diarrhoea. *Trans. Bombay Med. Congress.*

MANNING, C. T. (1907). *Psilosis Pigmentosa. Report to the Government of Barbados.*

MANSON, PATRICK (1880). Notes on Sprue. *China Imper. Marit. Customs Med. Rep.* 19th issue, 33.

—— (1909). *Tropical Diseases.* London. 5th edit.

MOORHEAD (1897). Psilosis or Sprue. *Indian Lancet*, X. 161.

MUSGRAVE (1902). Sprue in Manila. *American Med.* III. 389, 429.

ROBSON, A. W. MAYO (1907). A Note on Interstitial Pancreatitis in its Relation to Sprue. *Brit. Med. Journ.* II. 203.

SQUIRE, MAURICE F. (1906). A Case of Sprue treated by Strawberries. *Lancet*, II. 1659.

STRAIN (1905). A Discussion on Sprue and Hill Diarrhoea. *Brit. Med. Journ.* II. 1285.

THIN, G. (1883). On a peculiar disease of Hot Climates (Psilosis Linguae—Psilosis Mucosae Intestini). *Practitioner*, XXXI. 169.

—— (1887). "Psilosis or Sprue": Its nature and treatment. *Ibid.* XXXIX. 337, 401.

—— (1890). Psilosis (Linguae et Mucosae Intestini). *Brit. Med. Journ.* I. 1357.

—— (1892). On the Symptoms and Pathology of Psilosis (linguae et intestini). *Med. Chir. Trans.* LXXV. 285.

—— (1897). *Psilosis or Sprue, its Nature and Treatment.* 2nd edit.

—— (1899). Discussion on Psilosis or Sprue. *Brit. Med. Journ.* II. 637.

—— (1899). A case of Psilosis cured by Strawberries and Milk. *Journ. Trop. Med.* II. 43.

TWINING (1835). *Clinical Illustrations of Diseases in Bengal.* 2nd edit.

WETHERED (1890-1). Psilosis or Sprue. *Trans. Path. Soc. Lond.* XLII. 116.

WIJEYSAKERE, W. (1904). Tabes Mesenterica and Ceylon Sore Mouth and Diarrhoea. *Journ. Trop. Med.* VII. 164.

WILLIAMS and SPENCER (1902). Note on a Case of Sprue. *Lancet*, II. 216.

YOUNG, E. H. (1903). Treatment of a Formidable Case of Sprue by Diet. *Lancet*, I. 873.

YOUNGE, G. H. (1905). Pepsin in Sprue and Hill Diarrhoea. *Brit. Med. Journ.* II. 1519.

English References to Hill Diarrhoea

BARRY, G. C. (1906). Notes on the Prevalence of Hill Diarrhoea. *Ind. Med. Gaz.* XLI. 132.

CHEEVERS, N. (1886). *The Diseases of India*, 574.

CROMBIE (1892). Hill Diarrhoea. *Ind. Med. Gaz.* XXVII. 129.

DUNCAN (1905). Hill Diarrhoea. *Brit. Med. Journ.* II. 1283.

FAYRER, J. (1893). Hill Diarrhoea, in Davidson's *Hygiene and Diseases of Warm Climates*, 521.

—— (1881). *Ibid. Tropical Dysentery and Chronic Diarrhoea*, 134.

GRANT (1854). Hill Diarrhoea and Dysentery. *Ind. Annals Med. Sci.* I. 311.

MACPHERSON (1887). Hill Diarrhoea and its Treatment. *Ind. Med. Gaz.* XXII. 193.

MAYNARD (1906). Hill Diarrhoea. *Brit. Med. Journ.* I. 141.

MOORE (1886). *Diseases of India.* 2nd edit. 167.

MORISON and CHITRE (1912). Causes of Diarrhoea in Poona. *India Sanitary Conference.*

NEATHERLY (1892). Treatment of Hill Diarrhoea. *Ind. Med. Gaz.* XXVII. 259.

French References to Sprue

BERENGER-FERAUD (1883). *Traité théoretique de la dysenterie.* Paris.

BERTRAND (1878). De la pancréatine dans la diarrhée chronique de Cochinchine. *Arch. de Méd. Nav.* XXIX. 352.

BERTRAND et FONTAN (1886-7). De l'entero-colite chronique endémique des pays chauds, diarrhée de Cochinchine. *Arch. de Méd. Nav.* XLV. 211 *et seq.* XLVI. 37 *et seq.*

CALMETTE (1893). Étude expérimentale de la dysenterie ou entero-colite endémique d'extrême Orient, et des abscès du foie d'origine dysenterique. *Arch. de Méd. Nav.* LX. 207.

CHAUVIN (1878). Anguillule stercorale dans la diarrhée des Antilles. *Arch. de Méd. Nav.* XXIX. 154.

JULIEN (1864). Aperçu sur les lésions anatomiques de la dysenterie en Cochinchine. *Thèse de Montpellier.*

KELSCH (1873). Anatomie pathologique de la diarrhée de Cochinchine. *Arch. de Physiol.* V. 687.

KELSCH et KIENER (1884). *Arch. de Physiol.* XVI. I. 186.

—— (1889). *Traité des maladies des pays chauds.* Paris.

LAVERAN (1877). Note relative au nématoide de la diarrhée de Cochinchine. *Gaz. hebd. de Méd.* 2me ser. XIII. 116.

LAYET (1877). Études d'hygiène intertropicale. *Arch. de Méd. Nav.* XXVII. 186.

LE DANTEC (1900). *Pathologie exotique.* Paris.

—— (1908). Présence d'une levure dans le Sprue. *Compt. Rend. de la Soc. de Biol.* LXIV. 1066. Also, *Bull. de la Soc. de Path. Exot.* I. 342.

NORMAND, A. (1877). Mémoire sur la diarrhée dite de Cochinchine. *Arch. de Méd. Nav.* XXVII. 35, and 102.

NORMAND, A. (1878). Rôle étiologique de l'anguillule dans la diarrhée de Cochinchine. *Arch. de Méd. Nav.* XXX. 214.

PORTE (1879). Indican dans l'urine de deux malades atteints de diarrhée de Cochinchine. *Arch. de Méd. Nav.* XXXI. 467.

ROUX (1889). *Traité pratique des maladies des pays chauds.* Paris.

TREILLE (1884). Note sur un bacille courbé de diarrhée de Cochinchine. *Arch. de Méd. Nav.* XLII. 229.

German References to Sprue

BOHNE, A. (1908). Ein Fall von Sprue und seine Behandlung. *Deutsch. med. Wochenschr.* XXVI. 1143.

BURG, VAN DER (1887). Vortrag a. d. 60 Vers. Deutsch. Naturf. und Aerzte, Wiesbaden. *Deutsche Kolonialzeitung*, 160.

FABER, K. (1904). Ein Fall chronischer Tropendiarrhoea (Sprue) mit anatomischer Untersuchung des Digestionstractus. *Archiv f. Verdauungskrankh.* IX. 333.

GRONEMAN, J. (1887). Das Tropenklima der Malayischen Inseln und seine Wirkung auf Europäer. *Deutsche Kolonialzeitung*, 439, 466.

HASPER, M. (1831). *Ueber die Natur und Behandlung der Krankheiten der Tropenländer*, I. 306. Leipzig.

HEYMANN (1855). *Versuch einer path.-therap. Darstellung der Krankheiten in den Tropenländern*, 70.

HIRSCH, A. (1886). *Handbuch der Hist.-geograph. Patholog.* 2nd edit. III. 173.

JUSTI, K. (1913). Beiträge zur Kenntnis der Sprue (Aphthae tropicae). Beiheft. *Archiv f. Schiffs- u. Tropen-Hyg.* XVII. Beiheft 10, 5–53.

KOHLBRUGGE (1901). Die Aetiologie der Aphthae Tropicae. *Archiv f. Schiffs- u. Tropen-Hyg.* V. 394.

LEEDE, C. ST. (1913). Ein Fall von Sprue durch Erdbeeren gebessert. *Zeitschr. f. Hyg. und Infektionskr.* LVII. 578–586.

MENSE, C. (1903). Ueber die Schwankungen des Rhodankaliumgehalts im Speichel. *Archiv f. Schiffs- und Tropen-Hyg.* VII. 325.

OEFELE, F. VON (1905). Kotzusammensetzung bei Aphthae Tropicae. *Janus*, X. 495.

RICHARTZ, H. (1905). Ueber Aphthae Tropicae oder Indische Sprue. *München. med. Wochenschr.* LII. 640.

ROSTOSKI (1909). Ueber chronische Tropendiarrhoe (Sprue). *München. med. Wochenschr.* LVI. 366.

SCHEUBE, B. (1903). *Die Krankheiten der warmen Länder.* 3rd edit. Jena.

VOGELIUS, F. (1905). Milchdiät bei chronischer Tropendiarrhöe. *Arch. f. Verdauungskr.* XV. 44.

WALTER, G. TH. (1905). Indische Spruw, Appendicitis larvata. *Nederl. Tijdsch. v. Geneesk.* XLI. pt. I. 854.

WEGELE, C. (1913). Ueber die diätetische Behandlung gewisser Formen chronischer Diarrhöe und speziell von "Indian Sprue." *Med. Klin.* IX. 866.

Dutch References to Sprue

BOSCH (1837). *Over de Indische Sprouw (Aphthae Orientales).* Amsterdam.

BURG, VAN DER (1880). *Indische Spruw (Aphthae tropicae).* Monograph. Batavia.

—— (1881). Indische Spruw. *Tijdschr. v. Geneesk. v. Ned. Ind.* 1881, I.

—— (1881). Vertaling van Manson's "Notes on Sprue." *Tijdschr. v. Geneesk. v. Ned. Ind.* 267.

116   *Researches on Sprue*

BURG, VAN DER (1887). *De Geneesheer in Nederl. Indië*, II. 609. Batavia.

—— (1890). Behandeling in Europa van zieken komende uit heete klimaat. *Tijdschr. v. Geneesk.* 145.

DOZY, J. P. (1876). *Geneesk. gids voor Nederl. Indië*, 91. Amsterdam.

FABER, KNUD (1904). Tijdfaelde of chronisch Tropendiarrhoe (Spruw), met anatomisch Undersogelse of Tordojelseskanalen. *Hospitalstidende*, XLVII. 313.

GREINER, C. G. (1859). Aphthae tropicae. *Geneesk. Tijdschr. v. Ned.-Ind.* VI. 15.

—— (1873). Aphthae tropicae. *Ibid.* III. 891.

HAAN DE, J. (1902). Indische Spruw. *Geneesk. Tijdschr. v. Ned. Indië*, XLII. No. 3, 311.

HAEFTEN, VAN F. W. (1902). Iets over het speeksel bij Ind. Spruw. *Geneesk. Tijdschr. v. Ned. Ind.* XLII. No. 4, 431.

KOHLBRUGGE, J. H. F. (1901). Eene bijdrage tot de aetiologie der Ind. Spruw. (Psilosis.) *Ned. Tijdschr. v. Geneesk.* II. No. 16.

—— (1902). Klin-Waarnemingen omtrent darmziekten in de tropen. (In *Talma's feestbundel.*)

MAURER, G. (1903). De aetiologie van beri-beri en psilosis. *Geneesk. Tijdschr. v. Ned. Ind.* XLIII. No. 6, 836.

RADEMAKER, JR. G. A. (1906). Onderzoekingen naar aanleiding van een Geval van Indische Spruw. *Dissertation.* Leiden.

SCHEER, VAN DER (1905). Aphthae tropicae. In *Handbuch der Tropenkrankheiten* von C. Mense, II. 1.

—— (1905). Indische Spruw. Een bijdrage tot de kenntis der appendicitis larvata. *Nederl. Tijdschr. v. Geneesk.* No. 10, 637.

SCHORRENBURG (1843–44). Geneeskundinge mededeelingen over de Indische Spruw. *Nederl. Lancet*, VI. 180.

SWAVING, C. (1864). Een bijdrage tot de Studie der Oost-Indische geneesmiddelen uit het plantenrijk. *Nederl. Tijdsch. v. Geneesk.*

References to Yeast Literature

BUSSE (1896). *Centralbl. f. Bakteriol.* XX. 236.

BUTLIN and SPENCER (1900). *Diseases of the Tongue.*

CALMETTE (1893). *Ann. Inst. Past.* VI. 604.

CAO (1900). *Ztschr. f. Hyg. u. Infectionskr.* XXXIV. 282–340.

FERMI and ARUCH (1895). *Centralbl. f. Bakteriol.* XVII. 593.

FISCHER and BREBECH (1894). *Zur Morphologie, Biologie und Systematik der Monilia candida.*

FOULERTON, A. G. R. (1900). *Journ. Path. and Bact.* VI. 37.

HANSEN (1893). *Centralbl. f. Bakteriol.* XIII. 16.

HIBLER (1904). *Ibid.* XXXVI. 505.

KLEIN (1901). Pathogénie. *Journ. of Hygiene*, I. 90.

—— (1902). *Centralbl. f. Bakteriol.* XXXI. 76.

LANGERHANS (1887). *Archiv f. Path. Anat.* CIX. 352.

PLAUT (1903). *Handbuch d. Path. Microorg.* Kolle und Wassermann, I. 575.

RETTGER (1904). *Centralbl. f. Bakteriol.* XXXVI. 519.

RONCALI (1895). *Ibid.* XVIII. 432.

SANFELICE (1895). *Ibid.* XVII. 625.

SCHMORL (1890). *Ibid.* VII. 329.

STERNBERG (1902). Ziegler's *Beitr. z. Path. Anat. und Allg. Path.* XXXII. 1.

STILL (1902). *Common Disorders and Diseases of Childhood.* 2nd edit., 218.
TOKISHIGE (1896). *Centralbl. f. Bakteriol.* XIX. 105.
VUILLEMIN (1898). *Compt. Rend. Hebd. Acad. Sci.* CXXVII. 630.

References to Pathology

BLOCH, C. E. (1903). Anatomische Untersuchungen über der Magen u. Darmkanal des Säuglings. *Jahrb. f. Kinderheilk.* LVIII. 121.

—— (1903). Studien über Magen-Darmkatarrh bei Säuglingen. *Jahrb. f. Kinderheilk.* 1903, LVIII. 733.

—— (1904). Die Säuglings-atrophie und die Panethischen Zellen. *Jahrb. f. Kinderheilk.* LIX. 1.

FABER and BLOCH (1900). Ueber die pathologischen Veränderungen der Digestionstraktus bei der perniciosen anaemiae und über die sogennante Darmatrophie. *Ztschr. f. Klin. Med.* XL. 98.

HUNTER (1909). *The Severest Anaemias.*

APPENDIX I

THE POPULATION OF CEYLON IN 1911[1]

Total population

Race	♂	♀
All races	2,175,030	1,931,320
Sinhalese	1,419,561	1,295,859
Tamils	570,049	488,968
Moors	148,386	118,239
Europeans	4645	2947
Burghers & Eurasians	13,341	13,322
Malays	6813	6177
Veddas	2792	2540
Others	9443	3278

Population all told, 4,106,350

Estate population

Province	No. of estates	Persons	Males	Females
Western	173	44,145	25,334	18,811
Central	958	279,317	148,767	130,550
Northern	6	202	115	87
Southern	47	9,486	5,694	3,792
North Western	156	15,006	9,412	5,594
Eastern	4	381	300	81
Uva	192	71,957	38,180	33,777
Sabaragamuwa	297	92,973	50,756	42,217
All Ceylon	1,833	513,467	278,558	234,909

Estate population by race

Province	All races		Sinhalese		Tamils		Moors		Europeans		Burghers and Eurasians		Malays		Others	
	♂	♀	♂	♀	♂	♀	♂	♀	♂	♀	♂	♀	♂	♀	♂	♀
Western	25,334	18,811	4,307	2,340	20,358	16,080	220	149	145	29	120	87	107	95	77	31
Central	148,767	130,550	8,446	5,004	136,362	122,435	1,707	1,500	942	506	449	382	330	305	531	418
Northern	115	87	0	0	113	86	0	0	2	1	0	0	0	0	0	0
Southern	5,694	3,792	2,279	1,115	3,267	2,594	42	31	33	4	29	15	1	0	43	33
Eastern	300	81	2	1	247	63	12	2	10	4	10	4	19	7	0	0
North Western	9,412	5,594	3,627	1,854	5,466	3,550	93	50	35	11	63	63	17	17	111	49
Uva	38,180	33,777	2,016	967	35,280	32,282	427	232	214	106	87	59	88	88	68	42
Sabaragamuwa	50,756	42,217	4,382	2,159	43,604	37,979	660	486	254	69	190	122	99	64	1,567	1,338
Total	278,558	234,909	25,059	13,440	244,697	215,069	3,161	2,450	1,635	730	948	732	661	576	2,397	1,911

[1] Taken from "The Census of Ceylon," 1911. E. B. Denham, F.R.S.S., Ceylon Civil Service.

APPENDIX II

THE NUMBER OF EUROPEANS RESIDENT IN THE DIFFERENT
PROVINCES

(exclusive of the military and shipping population)

Province	♂	♀	Total
Western	2047	1237	3284
Central	1537	1142	2679
Northern	96	60	156
Southern	157	116	273
Eastern	68	43	111
North Western	95	52	147
Uva	322	194	516
North Central	24	12	36
Sabaragamuwa	299	91	390
Total in all Ceylon	4645	2947	7592

Colombo district and municipality (Western Province)

	♂	♀	Total
Municipality	1685	1067	2752
District	222	137	359

Total, 3111 in Colombo district and municipality.

APPENDIX III

TEMPERATURE AND RAINFALL

Average monthly mean temperature of stations in Ceylon

Province	Station	Jan.	Feb.	March	April	May	June	July	Aug.	Sept.	Oct.	Nov.	Dec.	For one year	Rainfall Amount for one year
Western	Colombo Observatory	79·1	79·6	80·6	82·3	82·9	81·8	80·5	80·6	80·9	79·8	79·2	78·8	80·5	59·67"
,,	Colombo Fort	79·1	80·2	82·1	82·6	82·3	81	80·5	80·7	80·7	80	79·8	79·1	80·7	45·69"
Sabaragamuwa	Ratnapura	70·0	79·3	80·4	80·5	80·4	79·4	79·4	79·3	79·1	79	78·1	80·1	79·4	128·04"
North Western	Puttalam	78·6	80·1	82·8	84·2	84·6	83·3	82·6	82·6	82·7	80·1	78·5	76	81·4	30·08"
North Central	Anuradhapura	73·3	78·3	81·5	82·6	82·9	80·4	82·4	82·5	82·4	80·2	78·1	76·4	80·3	53·81"
Northern	Mannar	78·6	79·8	82·3	84·9	85·3	84·1	82·8	82·6	82·6	81·7	79·8	78·2	81·9	33·34"
,,	Jaffna	78	79·6	85·6	85·5	84·9	86·6	82·7	82·4	83·5	81·4	79·1	77·5	82·1	43·70"
Eastern	Trincomalee	77·7	81·2	81·3	83·4	84·4	83·8	83·1	82·7	82·3	80·7	78·8	77·6	81·4	74·78"
,,	Batticaloa	76·6	77·7	79·8	82	83	83·4	82·9	82·2	81·8	80·2	78·3	76·6	80·4	70·19"
Southern	Hambantota	78·2	79·2	85	81·6	81·3	80·5	80·4	80·3	80·1	79·9	79	78·5	80	32·91"
,,	Galle	78	79·3	81·1	81·7	81·4	80·3	79·7	79·8	79·9	79·3	78·9	78·1	79·8	80·99"
Central	Kandy	73·5	75·1	77·4	77·5	78·5	75·6	74·9	75	74·9	75·2	75·1	73·4	75·5	81·09"
,,	Nuwara Eliya	56·8	57·8	60·7	60·3	60·9	58·3	57·4	57·9	58·1	58·4	57·9	57·3	58·5	96·34"
,,	Hakgala	57·3	58·4	60·6	62·2	63·2	60·9	60·1	61·6	60·8	60·4	59·2	57·4	60·2	107·15"
Uva	Badulla	69·4	71	73	74·9	75·4	75·2	74·7	74·8	74·4	73·7	71·9	70·4	73·2	75·73"
,,	Diyatalawa	63·9	65·6	67·6	68·8	70·1	69·7	69·1	69·1	68·8	67·3	65·7	62·2	67·5	73·77"
North Western	Kurunegala	77·5	78·7	82·4	82·3	82·1	80·2	79·7	79·8	80	79·2	68·6	77·4	79·8	67·08"

APPENDIX IV

CLINICAL ACCOUNT OF CASES OF SPRUE IN NATIVES

(1) Moor male, aged 16. Seen in the General Hospital, Colombo. Important points in this case as follows: incessant frothy diarrhoea; no ankylostome ova in the stools; oedema of extremities; intense anaemia. Hb. 40 per cent., rbc. 1,900,000, poikilocytosis; smooth sore tongue covered with a slimy growth of thrush fungus; liver small to percussion, haemic murmur over the base of the heart. Death six days after first examination; no post-mortem permitted.

(2) Sinhalese male, aged 35. Seen in the General Hospital, Colombo. Incessant and frothy diarrhoea; a few ankylostome ova found; extreme emaciation; smooth sore tongue; cracked raw areas at angles of mouth; buccal cavity covered with a slimy growth of thrush; oedema of both feet; oedema of bases of both lungs. Anaemia, Hb. 70 per cent., rbc. 3,500,000, no poikilocytosis. Death ten days after; only partial post-mortem permitted.

(3) Tamil female, aged 30. Seen at Nuwara Eliya Hospital. Frothy diarrhoea; no ankylostome ova in the stools; emaciation extreme; tongue raw and sore; liver dulness diminished to percussion. Anaemia, Hb. 70 per cent., rbc. 3,300,000.

(4) Sinhalese female, aged 37, had been treated by Dr Drummond for several years for a chronic diarrhoea characterised by pale and frothy stools; tongue red and sore but had improved under treatment; when I saw her symptoms were in abeyance, no ankylostome ova were found in the stools.

(5) Sinhalese female, aged 40. Seen in Lady Havelock Hospital, Colombo. Is said to have had a chronic but intermittent diarrhoea for eight years; mouth very sore; tongue glazed; raw and bleeding areas at the angles of the mouth overgrown with a slimy growth of thrush; abdomen distended; liver dulness much diminished to percussion. Anaemia marked, Hb. 50 per cent., rbc. 2,075,000; the stools contained a few ankylostome ova.

(6) Sinhalese male, aged 26. Seen in the General Hospital, Colombo. Frothy diarrhoea; oedema of the feet; great emaciation; tongue smooth and painful, covered with a slimy growth of thrush; liver dulness diminished to percussion; abdomen distended; a few ankylostomes in the stools. Death a fortnight later; only a limited post-mortem permitted.

(7) Sinhalese male, aged 53. Seen in the General Hospital, Colombo. Incessant frothy diarrhoea; tongue smooth and very sore; oedema of both legs; area of liver dulness diminished to percussion; abdomen distended. Anaemia, Hb. 80 per cent., rbc. 2,600,000. Great numbers of yeast cells and ankylostome ova found in the stools.

(8) Sinhalese female, aged 34, living in good circumstances in Kandy. Had sprue symptoms—sore tongue and diarrhoea before childbirth. Five weeks after birth of child symptoms became acute. Tongue very sore; fungiform papillae very red and prominent; aphthae situated on the hard palate and cheeks; flatulence; dyspepsia; oesophageal and rectal pain marked; distension of abdomen; oedema of both legs; great anaemia. Area of liver dulness diminished to percussion; haemic basal cardiac murmur. Stools frothy light cream coloured contained ova

of *Trichocephalus dispar*, but no ankylostomes. Death occurred three weeks later; no post-mortem permitted.

(9) Sinhalese female, aged 28. Seen a fortnight after childbirth in the Lady Havelock Hospital, Colombo, with a history of sore mouth of two months duration; constant diarrhoea; tongue red and smooth covered with patches of thrush; very anaemic and emaciated; abdominal distension marked. Stools contained ova of *Trichocephalus dispar*; but no ankylostomes.

(10) Tamil male, aged 35; seen in Jaffna. Constant diarrhoea, very emaciated and anaemic; abdomen distended; liver dulness diminished to percussion; haemic cardiac murmur. Tongue raw, red and smooth. A few ankylostome ova found in the stools. Death six weeks later; post-mortem permitted, tissues obtained for section.

(11) Tamil boy aged 8; seen in Batticaloa, Eastern Province. History of sore mouth and tongue; constant diarrhoea; stools large, pale and frothy; unable to eat anything but milk and rice. A bare patch on dorsum of tongue; fungiform papillae red and prominent; distension of abdomen; emaciated and slightly anaemic, Hb. 70 per cent. Death three weeks later; no post-mortem permitted.

APPENDIX V

DETAILS OF VARIOUS ESTATE BUNGALOWS AND THEIR RELATION TO SPRUE

Total of 143 Returns

CENTRAL PROVINCE

In the Central Province 98 returns were submitted as follows:

Estates 98 = 78 tea; 15 tea and rubber; 4 rubber; 1 mixed cultivation.

    36 bungalows were built of wood;

    28 of these contained dry rot;

    16 were considered unhealthy. (Nature of illness recorded below.)

Illness considered with regard to condition of bungalow, rainfall and altitude

Illness	Industry	Age of bungalow	Rainfall	Altitude
Sprue (1 case)	Tea	20 years	120″	2100 ft.
„ „	Tea	25 „	180″	4500 „
„ „	Tea	25 „	84″	4700 „
„ „ chronic diarrhoea (1 case)	Tea	30 „	100″	4000 „
„ „ „ „ „	Tea	30 „	90″	3500 „
„ „ „ „ (several)	Tea	30 „	115″	4300 „
„ „ „ „ (1 case)	Tea	60 „	130″	2700 „
„ „ sore throats (several)	Tea	20 „	120″	4500 „
Headaches and sore throats	Tea	35 „	108″	4300 „
Morning diarrhoea	Tea	40 „	110″	4000 „
Diarrhoea and sore throats	Tea	45 „	130″	4500 „
Sore throats	Tea	42 „	130″	4400 „
Diarrhoea, nausea, drowsiness	Tea	35 „	130″	5300 „
Diarrhoea and sore throats	Tea	35 „	120″	4500 „
Sore throats	Tea	Very old	160″	2600 „
Diarrhoea and headaches	Tea	5 „	130″	5000 „

Unhealthy without dry rot

One case of sprue occurred in a wooden bungalow 38 years old; no "dry rot." Rainfall 115"; altitude 4300 ft.

Of the 62 other bungalows in this province (built of wattle and daub, brick or stone):

20 contained "dry rot" in the timbers;
6 of these were said to be unhealthy.

Illness			Industry	Bungalow built of		Age of bungalow	Rainfall	Altitude
1 Sprue case	..	..	Tea	Wattle and daub		40 years	100"	4800 ft.
"	"	..	..	"	"	"	30 "	90"	5000 "
"	"	..	..	"		Brick	15 "	90"	3200 "
"	"	..	.. Tea and rubber	"		41 "	140"	200 "
Sore throats	..	..	Tea	"		35 "	90"	5000 "
Diarrhoea and drowsiness			"	"		12 "	195"	4100 "

3 others were said to be unhealthy, but contained no "dry rot."

Illness			Industry	Bungalow built of	Age of bungalow	Rainfall	Altitude
1 Sprue case	..	..	Tea	Stone	new	240"	4000 ft.
1 Sprue case (16 years ago)			Tea and rubber	,,	40 years	132"	2500 "
Sore tongue	..	..	Tea	"	?	119"	4100 "

PROVINCE OF SABARAGAMUWA

Estates 17 = 3 tea, 4 rubber, 10 tea and rubber.

8 bungalows were built of wood;
1 (only) contained dry rot (healthy).

The only case of ill-health in the 17 returns from this province was as follows
1 case of chronic diarrhoea; stone bungalow (age not given); no "dry rot."
Tea estate: rainfall 150"; altitude 3500 feet.

PROVINCE OF UVA

Estates 16 = 9 tea, 2 rubber, 5 tea and rubber.

3 bungalows were built of wood;
2 of them were said to be unhealthy.

Illness			Industry	Age of bungalow	Rainfall	Altitude
1 sprue case	..	.. .. Tea and rubber		20 years	75"	3200 ft.
Sore throats and headaches	..		Tea	70 .,	85"	4000 "

4 other bungalows contained "dry rot";
1 was said to be unhealthy.

Illness	Built of	Industry	Age of bungalow	Rainfall	Altitude
Chronic diarrhoea (1 case) ..	Modern wattle	Tea	30 years	100"	3500 ft.

EASTERN PROVINCE

There was only one return submitted from this Province, from a coconut estate; the bungalow was built of brick and was considered healthy.

WESTERN PROVINCE

Estates 10 = 4 rubber, 6 tea and rubber.
  4 bungalows were built of wood;
  1 contained "dry rot" (healthy).
  Of the other 6 one contained "dry rot," this was said to be unhealthy.

Illness	Built of	Industry	Age of bungalow	Rainfall	Altitude
Diarrhoea	Brick	Tea and rubber	20	150″	200 ft.

NORTH WESTERN PROVINCE

Only one return was submitted, from a mixed tea and rubber estate; the bungalow was built of brick and considered healthy.

APPENDIX VI

A LIST OF CEYLON MOSQUITOES
(as identified by Col. Alcock, C.I.E., F.R.S.)

(E.P., S.P., *denote abbreviations for Eastern, Southern Province, etc.*)

(1) ANOPHELINES.

Species	Where procured from
Anopheles (*Myzomyia*) *rossii* Giles.	Badulla (Uva) [2300 ft.] Nuwara Eliya (C.P.) [6600 ft.], Kurunegala (N.W.P.) [320 ft.], Batticaloa (E.P.) [sea-level].
„ „ *albirostris* Theob.	Kurunegala [320 ft.].
„ „ *culifacies* Giles.	„
„ „ *punctulata* Donitz.	„ and Badulla [2200 ft.].
„ (*Myzorhynchus*) *sinensis* Wied.	„
„ „ *barbirostris* V. de Wulp.	„
„ (*Nyssorhynchus*) *fuliginosus* Giles.	„
„ „ *jamesi* Theob.	„
„ „ *maculatus* Theob.	Nuwara Eliya and Kurunegala.
Anopheles gigas var. *refutans*[1], new sp. Alcock.	Nuwara Eliya.

[1] *refutans* resembles *gigas* except that the palps have three or four very narrow light tawny bands, one of which is situated at the tip.

(2) CULICINES.

Species	Where procured from
Culex concolor	Kurunegala and Colombo (W.P.).
„ *gelidus*	Tangalla (S.P.), Kurunegala and Colombo.
„ *mimeticus*	Nuwara Eliya. Kurunegala.
„ *fatigans*	Badulla, Kurunegala, Tangalla and Nuwara Eliya.
„ *vishnui*	Weligama (S.P.), Muttur (E.P.), Tangalla and Badulla.
„ *fuscocephala*	Tangalla, Badulla and Nuwara Eliya.
Culicomyia ceylonica	Badulla and Nuwara Eliya.
Schlerotatus pallidostriatus	Tissa (S.P.) and Kurunegala.
„ *stenoetrus*	Weligama (S.P.).
Desvoidea obturbans	Anuradhapura (N.W.P.) and Kurunegala.
Mansonioides uniformis	Kanthalai (E.P.), Chilaw (N.W.P.) [sea-level], Talawa (N.P.), Tissa, Weligama, Hakmana and Illekmulla (S.P.).
„ *annulifer*	Tissa (S.P.).
Aedes mediofasciatus	Matara (S.P.).
Stegomyia scutellaris	Peradeniya (C.P.) [1800 ft.].
„ *sugens*	Peradeniya.
„ *trilineata*	Ramboda (C.P.) [5000 ft.].

(3) CORETHRINAE.

Corethra asiatica	Vavuniya (N.P.).

APPENDIX VII

Table showing incidence of sore sprue-like tongues in natives. All natives examined in hospitals and gaols where a representative collection of local inhabitants was found

Province	TAMILS No. examined	TAMILS Sore tongues With diarrhoea	TAMILS Sore tongues No diarrhoea	TAMILS With obvious ankylostomiasis	SINHALESE No. examined	SINHALESE Sore tongues With diarrhoea	SINHALESE Sore tongues No diarrhoea	SINHALESE With obvious ankylostomiasis	MOORS No. examined	MOORS Sore tongues With diarrhoea	MOORS Sore tongues No diarrhoea	MOORS With obvious ankylostomiasis
Uva	78♂ 34♀	1♂ 2♀	5♀ 2♀	—	4♂	—	4♂	—				
E.P.	33♂ 13♀	—	6♀	—	17♂ 4♀	—	7♂	—	3♂	—		
N.W.P.	31♂	—	—	—	173♂ 27♀	—	2♂	—	1♂	—		
C.P.	21♀	1♀ 1♂	1♀ 11♀	1♂ 3♀	30♂ 16♀	2♂	—	—	1♂	—		
W.P.	159♂ 122♀ 31♂	—	5♀ 1♂	—	130♂ 37♀	—	19♂ 3♀ 1♂ 1♀	—	15♂	—	5♂	
Sab.	22♂ 14♀	—	1♂ 1♀	—	12♀ 7♂	—	—	—				
S.P.	25♂ 12♀	—	5♀	—	188♂ 31♀	—	29♂ 5♀	—	9♂	—	1♂	
N.P.	37♂ 28♀	1♂	—	1♂								
Total	**660**	**6**	**38**	**5**	**576**	**2**	**71**	**0**	**29**	**0**	**6**	**0**

1265 examined; 128 had sore tongues

Incidence of sore tongues in gaols with inmates from various parts of the island

Name of gaol	TAMILS No. examined	TAMILS With diarrhoea	TAMILS No diarrhoea	TAMILS With obvious ankylostomiasis	SINHALESE No. examined	SINHALESE With diarrhoea	SINHALESE No diarrhoea	SINHALESE With obvious ankylostomiasis	MOORS No. examined	MOORS With diarrhoea	MOORS No diarrhoea	MOORS With obvious ankylostomiasis
Jaffna, N.P.	38♂	—	7♂	—	128♂	—	37♂	—	18♂	—	6♂	—
Anuradhapura, N.C.P.	6♂ 6♀	—	1♂ 2♀	—								
Total	**50**	**0**	**10**	**0**	**128**	**0**	**37**	**0**	**18**	**0**	**6**	**0**

196 examined; 53 had sore tongues. Of the total number examined in Ceylon (1461) 181 had smooth tongues.

APPENDIX VIII

Results of 37 Wassermann (Noguchi) reactions

Nos. examined	Condition of tongue	Reaction	
3	Completely smooth	3 –	
5	„ „ with superficial fissures	2 –	3 +
5	Fissured with enlarged fungiform papillae	5 –	
6	Completely smooth	4 –	2 +
5	Bare at tip and fissured	5 –	
3	Enlarged fungiform papillae	3 –	
4	Bare patches	4 –	
6	Normal tongues (as controls)	6 –	
37		32 –	5 +

The above cases were taken from patients suffering from sore tongues (with exceptions of 6 normals), inmates of Kandy, Dikoya Hospitals, and Welikadde Gaol, Colombo.

Noguchi's modification of the Wassermann was used throughout. Text-book methods were adhered to with the exception of the quantities of reagents employed.

These were as follows:

Washed red blood corpuscles	..	0·2 c.c.
Complement	..	0·025 c.c.
Antigen	..	0·1 c.c.
Patients and syphilitic sera ..	..	0·05 c.c. (inactivated at 56° C. ½ hr.)

Amboceptor (papers 5 mm. square containing each 1 drop of antihuman amboceptor, titre 1 : 800).

APPENDIX IX

*Table showing the relationship between the amount of fluid and proteid ingested
and the amount of urine and urea excreted in two cases of sprue*

			INGESTED			EXCRETED		
(I)								
Date		Total weight of food	Amount of fluid	Estimated proteid content of food	Approximate urea equivalent of food proteid	Amount of urine excreted	Amount of urea excreted	Weight of stool
May	15/12	2693 grammes	2244 c.c.	89 grammes	29·37 grammes	2300 c.c.	18·9 grammes	336 grammes
	16	,,	,,	,,	,,	2150	21·5	224
	17	2805	,,	99	33	3000	19·5	315
	18	,,	,,	,,	,,	2000	20·0	218
	29	2237	1018	90·75	29·9	3150	25·2	294
	30	,,	,,	,,	,,	1750	19·25	Nil
	31	,,	,,	,,	,,	1700	18·7	336
June	1/12	,,	,,	,,	,,	1350	18·9	96
	5	,,	,,	,,	,,	1400	16·8	112
	6	,,	,,	,,	,,	1300	16·9	Nil
	7	,,	,,	,,	,,	1200	19·2	196
	8	,,	,,	,,	,,	1350	20·25	Nil
(II)								
Aug.	25/12	1736	1698	67·9	22·41	2000	20·0	448
	26	2020	1981	79·24	26·15	1100	23·1	140
	27	2304	2264	90·56	29·8	1500	30·0	112
	28	2584	2547	101·8	33·6	1800	37·8	280
	29	,,	,,	,,	,,	1450	26·1	364
	30	2938	2830	113	37·3	2000	28·0	448
	31	3222	3113	124	41	1750	22·75	336
Sept.	2/12	,,	,,	,,	,,	2300	23·0	168
	3	,,	,,	,,	,,	2550	25·5	560
	4	,,	,,	,,	,,	2200	24·2	448
	5	2706	2264	90·56	29·8	2450	24·5	504
	6	2818	,,	,,	,,	1500	22·5	168

APPENDIX X

BLOOD COUNTS

Blood counts in European cases of sprue with active symptoms

Sex	Ova in stools	Duration of symptoms	Red cells	White cells	Haemoglobin	Polymorphs	Lymphocytes	Mononuclears	Eosinophiles	Remarks
♀	Nil	2¾ years	5,000,000	5,928	70 %	56 %	33 %	4 %	7 %	
♀	,,	7 ,,	5,000,000	6,552	100	58	35	5	2	
♂	,,	3 ,,	4,500,000	11,230	100	54	40	4	2	Fatal case
♀	,,	4 months	4,025,000	5,250	80	49	45	6	0	
♂	,,	9 ,,	3,975,000	—	90	—	—	—	—	
♂	,,	4 years	3,278,000	6,800	90	47	50	2	1	
♀	,,	6 months	3,125,000	3,744	90	58	37	2	3	Fatal case
♂	,,	2 years	3,000,000	—	90	—	—	—	—	
♂	,,	6 months	2,925,000	4,056	90	54	41	4	1	
♂	,,	7 ,,	2,700,000	8,700	65	53	40	5	2	
♂	,,	3 years	2,000,000	10,000	70	42	55	2	1	
♀	,,	10 months	1,475,000	—	30	—	—	—	—	Fatal case
♀	,,	8 ,,	1,300,000	5,300	35	37	47	16	⅓	Fatal case

Sprue in natives

Sex	Ova in stools	Duration of symptoms	Red cells	White cells	Haemoglobin	Polymorphs	Lymphocytes	Mononuclears	Eosinophiles	Remarks
Sinhalese ♀	Nil	?	5,000,000	—	100 %	48 %	44 %	4 %	4 %	
,, ♂	Few ankylostomes	?	3,525,000	6552	70	59	40	1	0	Fatal case
Tamil ♀	Nil	?	3,312,000	7488	70	63	30	2	5	
,, ♂	Ankylostomes +	?	2,975,000	7488	60	83	13	0	4	
Sinhalese ♀	,,	?	2,275,000	7800	50	77	18	5	0	
Moor ♂	Nil	?	1,900,000	6240	40	65	32	3	0	Fatal case
Sinhalese ♂	Nil	?	1,633,000	3744	40	44	49	6	1	Fatal case

A. *Incomplete sprue without tongue symptoms*

♂	Nil	3 years	5,000,000	8112	100 %	46 %	46 %	5 %	3 %	
♀	,,	5 ,,	3,950,000	4056	80	40	53	5	2	
♂	,,	1 year	3,400,000	—	90	46	44	7	3	

B. *Incomplete sprue. (Chronic diarrhoea cases)*

Sex	Ova in stools	Duration of symptoms	Red cells	White cells	Haemoglobin	Polymorphs	Lymphocytes	Mononuclears	Eosinophiles	Remarks
♂	Nil	4 months	5,000,000	5,616	70 %	40 %	51 %	8 %	1 %	
♂	,,	2 years	5,000,000	5,616	100	60	33	5	3	
♂	,,	1 year	5,000,000	8,736	100	60	33	7	0	
♀	,,	3 months	5,000,000	6,552	100	68	27	3	2	
♀	,,	3 years	4,500,000	—	85	—	—	—	—	
♂	,,	2 ,,	4,200,000	10,296	100	58	33	8	1	
♂	,,	4 ,,	4,075,000	5,616	90	30	56	4	1	

Europeans who had apparently recovered from sprue

Sex	Ova in stools	No sprue symptoms noted for	Red cells	White cells	Haemo-globin	Differential blood count				Remarks
						Poly-morphs	Lympho-cytes	Mono-nuclears	Eosino-philes	
♂	Nil	1½ years	5,000,000	10,290	90 %	49 %	38 %	4 %	9 %	
♂	,,	1½ ,,	5,000,000	12,160	100	66	32	1	1	
♂	,,	1½ ,,	5,000,000	6,240	100	—	—	—	—	
♀	,,	2 ,,	4,500,000	—	95	42	55	2	1	
♂	,,	7 ,,	4,000,000	5,616	100	61	35	3	1	

Cases of amoebic dysentery for comparison

Sex	Ova in stools	Duration of symptoms	Red cells	White cells	Haemo-globin	Poly-morphs	Lympho-cytes	Mono-nuclears	Eosino-philes
♂	Nil	18 months	5,000,000	6,240	80 %	59 %	26 %	6 %	9 %
♂	,,	5 years	5,000,000	—	100	—	—	—	—
♀	,,	5 ,,	4,800,000	—	100	—	—	—	—
♂	,,	2 ,,	3,600,000	—	100	—	—	—	—
♂	,,	5 ,,	3,500,000	7,170	85	40	48	8	4

APPENDIX XI

DETAILS OF SPRUE CASES AND POST-MORTEMS

Sprue post-mortem A.

A single woman aged 36, of white parentage and born in Colombo, was first seen in April 1912.

History of the patient. In 1911 she went to Perth, W. Australia, where she stayed for three months. Sprue symptoms apparently commenced on board the boat on the return voyage; previous to this she had never suffered from any bowel complaint.

Her illness commenced with diarrhoea; the evacuations were especially frequent during the night-time and were painless. After a short time tongue symptoms and an excessive salivation were noted, though at times she complained of a feeling of dryness in the mouth and throat especially during the early hours of the morning.

Whilst in Colombo she was dieted on fruit and milk, but as her condition showed no signs of improvement, she was sent to Nuwara Eliya in May 1912 for special treatment. There was nothing in her previous history calling for comment. Her katamenia had ceased for eleven months and there was no history of syphilis.

Condition in May 1912. She was greatly emaciated and weighed only 119 lbs. Her abdomen was flaccid, the area of liver dulness normal; a basal systolic cardiac murmur was present. There was no actual diarrhoea, but her stools were large, light brown and pasty and coated with a considerable amount of mucus. The mouth symptoms were well marked, the whole of the buccal mucous membrane was inflamed, especially at the opening of Stenson's duct; several of her teeth were decayed, but there were no signs of pyorrhoea. The tip of the tongue was red, and the fungiform papillae inflamed and prominent. In scrapings made from the inflamed area yeast cells could be demonstrated microscopically in the superficial squamous epithelial cells. Anaemia was not marked, the red cells numbered 3,600,000 and haemoglobin was 90 per cent. The stools contained no parasitic ova. Urobilin could be demonstrated in the urine which was otherwise normal.

On milk and bael fruit treatment her condition much improved and the inflammation of the tongue and mouth rapidly subsided. After a month treatment was discontinued. She remained well subsequently for a time, but was eventually lost sight of till March 1913 when I found her in the General Hospital, Colombo.

Condition in March 1913. The patient was almost unrecognisable, every trace of subcutaneous fat had disappeared and she was reduced to a mere skeleton. The abdomen was sunken, there was oedema of the left ankle and numerous petechiae on the abdomen and legs. The skin was of a sallow yellow colour. There was incontinence of evil-smelling, liquid and dark grey faeces. The tongue was completely devoid of papillae and covered with yellowish-coloured crescentic patches of thrush. Death occurred on March 30th, 1913.

Post-mortem. The autopsy was commenced within two hours of death. It was not possible to weigh the body. No trace of subcutaneous or body fat was present; the muscles were of a dark brown colour.

Thorax. The thoracic cavity contained no free fluid.

Lungs. R. lung weighed 12 ozs., L. lung 9 ozs., both were very pale and oedematous; hypostatic pneumonic patches were present at the bases. Trachea, bronchi, thyroid gland and bronchial lymphatic glands were normal.

Heart. 3¾ ozs., flabby, ventricular walls thin, muscle very dark brown in colour (brown atrophy), the fluid and bright red blood did not show signs of great anaemia, the haemoglobin percentage being 80.

Digestive tract. Tongue dry, perfectly smooth and devoid of all papillae. Oesophagus was covered throughout its whole extent by a yellow diphtheritic membrane which when scraped off left a raw apparently granulating surface underneath. The stomach was contracted and contained no food, the mucous membrane which was coated with a layer of ropy mucus appeared otherwise normal.

Intestines. External appearances. There was no free fluid in the abdominal cavity. The jejunum was dark purple and congested especially on the peritoneal surface. The ileum was distended and transparent; the large intestine was contracted.

Internal appearances of the small intestine. No intestinal contents, save a few milk clots in the rectum, were found throughout the whole length of the intestinal canal, which was also coated with a thick layer of mucus as in the case of the stomach.

The duodenum and upper part of the jejunum were apparently normal, but the lower part of the jejunum was inflamed and of a cherry-red colour. The walls of the ileum, especially within two feet of the iliocaecal valve, appeared to be attenuated, and were transparent enough to allow large print to be easily read through them. Peyer's patches were quite normal and there were no signs of ulceration in the gut. The small veins in the submucosa were of large size and engorged with blood, thus giving the mucous membrane a stippled appearance. The thick mucus covering the ileum was bile-stained. The appendix was normal.

Internal appearances of the large intestine. The mucous membrane of the caecum was cherry-red in colour and covered with bile-stained mucus. The ascending colon appeared to be perfectly healthy. The transverse, descending, sigmoid pelvic colons and rectum were also coated with bile-stained mucus; the mucous membrane was of a cherry-red colour and had a rough appearance. The coats of the large intestine did not appear to be attenuated at all. No intestinal parasites were found.

The great and small omenta were completely devoid of fat.

Liver. 25 ozs., yellowish-brown in colour and friable; a fine interlobular fibrosis was visible. The gall-bladder was normal in size and full of dark green bile.

Spleen. 1¾ ozs., tough and dark, the capsule was marked by some minute granular thickenings.

Both the liver and spleen gave a positive iron reaction. (Potassium ferrocyanide and hydrochloric acid test.)

Pancreas. 1½ ozs., apparently quite normal.

Kidneys. R. 3 ozs., L. 3¼ ozs., dark in colour but otherwise normal.

In addition to these organs, the lymphatic glands, the salivary glands—sublingual, parotid and submaxillary,—the bladder, uterus and appendages, suprarenals, mesenteric arteries and veins, the inferior vena cava, etc. were examined and found to be to all external appearances normal.

The bone-marrow of the sternum was dark brown in colour.

Yeast cells and mycelium (*monilia*) were found in numbers in smears made from the tongue, oesophagus (the false membrane of which was formed almost entirely of these organisms), stomach, duodenum, jejunum, ileum, caecum, transverse colon, sigmoid colon and rectum, but none were found in smears made from the heart, liver, spleen, pancreas and gall-bladder.

Cultures were made by means of a syringe from all the main organs and inoculated into glucose-agar and glucose nutrient broth. Similar cultures were made from the mucus lining the intestinal canal by means of a platinum scraper; from these yeast cells were cultivated in 4 per cent. glucose-broth in great numbers throughout the whole length of the intestinal canal and from the kidney substance, but cultures from heart-blood, spleen and liver remained sterile.

Microscopical sections. All tissues were preserved in 4 per cent. formalin, cut in paraffin and stained by a number of methods which I will here briefly enumerate; so as to prevent repetition this statement applies to all the sections I shall describe,—haematoxylin and eosin, haematoxylin and van Gieson, Weigert, Giemsa, carbol-thionin, carbol·fuchsin decolourised by acid-alcohol, Heidenhain's iron haematoxylin and Levaditi.

Alimentary canal. In sections cut through various portions of the tongue the surface epithelium was vacuolated and stained badly, and in places covered with dead and desquamated stratified cells. On the cross-section of the tongue no papillae are visible. In certain areas where desquamation appears to have proceeded further than in others, the underlying corium of the papillae shows local accumulations of leucocytes, round cells and plasma cells and congestion of the capillary vessels. There are no evidences of a corresponding tissue reaction in the deeper strata of the tongue. In sections stained by Weigert's method yeast cells are seen growing into the desquamated epithelium; in some situations the mycelium is growing vertically, in others in a horizontal direction between the cells of the epithelial layer. Sections through the tip of the organ show that the desquamation of epithelium and yeast infiltration are found on both the dorsum and the under-surface. In sections stained by carbol thionin many other organisms can be distinguished in the dead epithelium, but not in the deeper intact tissues. In the epithelial cells invaded by penetrating mycelium numerous Gram-positive granules, possibly of keratohyaline, could be distinguished.

Buccal mucous membrane (palate and lower lip). There is vacuolation of the more superficial stratified epithelial cells which are being cast off. In certain papillae where the desquamation is complete there are local accumulations of leucocytes. In Weigert sections no yeast cells or mycelium can be seen penetrating the stratified epithelium.

Oesophagus. The stratified epithelial cells are vacuolated and evidently degenerated. The surface of the section has a ragged appearance where the desquamated cells are in the process of being cast off; the nuclei of these cells have undergone chromatolysis. In places there are patches of dead and desquamated epithelium still adhering to the surface which is infiltrated by yeast cells and mycelium growing vertically downwards. The mucous coat shows subacute inflammatory changes such as perivascular round-cell infiltration, capillary congestion, etc. The muscular coats appear normal.

Stomach. The columnar epithelium is preserved and the gastric glands appear normal. There are a few Russell's bodies in the inter-glandular tissue. No organisms or yeast cells can be made out within the mucosa.

Duodenum. There are numerous evidences of chronic irritation, such as congestion of the capillaries of the mucosa, perivascular infiltration in the submucosa, marked round-cell infiltration in the interstitial tissue and numerous hyaline Russell's bodies. The surface epithelium is preserved. No organisms can be seen in stained sections in the surface epithelium or in the deeper layers.

Jejunum. (*Two sections.*) The changes are similar to those found in the duodenum, but they are more intense and in addition the glandular epithelial cells are vacuolated and degenerated; capillary dilatation is marked. No organisms can be seen in the mucosa.

Ileum. (*Three sections.*) Much attention has been paid to the microscopic changes in this portion of the intestinal canal. Sections have been taken especially from areas wherever such macroscopic changes as decolouration of the surface and dilatation of the submucous vessels had been noted; the following is a summary of the changes found.

The majority of the villi are preserved, but in certain sections there are areas where only a small covering of mucous membrane can be seen. Where villi are present in the section they are much shrunken and irregular in shape (as noted by Justi). In most sections the surface epithelium is intact, the goblet cells are distended and there are many evidences of a chronic irritation, such as distension of the capillaries of the villi, the infiltration of the interstitial tissue with plasma cells, round cells and leucocytes. An invasion of the glandular tissue of the crypts also by leucocytes and round cells probably denoting a chronic inflammation of these structures can be seen, as was also noted by Justi in his case. There is a great increase in the fibrous elements in the submucosa where also the nutrient vessels are also greatly congested, in some cases to an extent as to fully occupy the whole submucous space; there is also a slight perivascular infiltration. No Russell's bodies are found in the mucous layer. Bacilli can be seen invading the mucosa only where a break of the surface has taken place evidently before death and where the surface epithelium is absent, and they are also found in small numbers in the lumen of the crypts. In some sections a few yeast cells can be distinguished in the mucosa.

Caecum. The surface epithelium is present in most sections and the goblet cells are distended with mucus. Large numbers of Russell's bodies as well as other evidences of a chronic irritation, as has just been noted in the ileum, are seen in the mucosa. In sections stained by carbol thionin numbers of organisms can be seen adhering to the epithelial surface and occasionally also situated within the lumen of the crypts. There is some round-cell infiltration in the submucosa. Here and there a budding yeast cell can be seen within the mucosa in Weigert-stained sections. The Panethian granules are well stained.

Transverse and sigmoid colons and rectum. The same histological changes are found in these tissues as in the caecum, so I need not recapitulate them. In thionin sections the surface epithelium and lumen of the crypts contain numbers of bacilli.

Organs. Heart. There is a large deposit of yellow-pigment granules in the cardiac muscle cells (as in brown atrophy). The capillaries are dilated and there are numbers of Russell's bodies in the interstitial tissue between the cardiac cells. Haemosiderin granules are present in small numbers.

Liver. There is extreme fatty degeneration of the liver cells at the periphery of the lobules and a large deposit of haemosiderin. Weigert and thionin stained sections show a number of rod-shaped bacilli and chains of streptococci in the larger bile ducts, and these are also invading the surrounding tissues.

Spleen. Sections of the spleen stained by haematoxylin and eosin show little but an increase of the trabecular tissue. The smaller veins in the trabeculae are dilated, and the pulp cells appear normal. In Weigert sections numbers of Gram-positive Russell's bodies, sometimes in clumps and chains, sometimes solitary, of a large size are in evidence. These bodies stain intensely red with weak carbol fuchsin and are not decolourised by acid-alcohol, but there are also numbers of small Gram-positive hyaline bodies in the swollen and evidently degenerated endothelial cells of the veins. Some of these cells are distended by these bodies almost to bursting point and their nuclei are degenerated; while others affected in this manner appear actually to have collapsed and to have scattered their contents into the blood stream. In unstained sections they appear as clear hyaline droplets but can be distinguished from the larger and acid-fast Russell's bodies by their lack of affinity for carbol fuchsin. These small bodies do not stain by haematoxylin, van Gieson or Levaditi's stain: they are distinctly eosinophile. With Marchi's stain they take on a light brown, with thionin blue and methol violet a deep blue, with Heidenhain's haematoxylin a deep black colour. In sections treated with iodine they appear as yellow, with Giemsa's stain as either blue, purple or pink globules. Their structure is homogeneous, though the appearance of a double contour which is sometimes obtained may be due to their refractile character.

A few granules of haemosiderin are found in the pulp cells.

Pancreas. There is marked post-mortem autodigestion; the secretory cells and the islands of Langerhans are normal, though there is an increase in the amount of interalveolar fibrous tissue.

Kidneys. Apparently normal.

Red bone-marrow. There is a marked absence of fat cells. In Giemsa-stained sections no abnormality in the normoblastic elements or in the fully formed erythrocytes can be seen, in this respect differing from similar sections in a case of pernicious anaemia with which they have been compared. In Weigert-stained sections clumps of hyaline Russell's bodies are seen lying free amongst the myelocytes.

Salivary glands, submaxillary, parotid and sublingual glands. Small collections of Russell's bodies were found in these tissues, but otherwise no other abnormal structures.

Lung. Section shows areas of hypostatic croupous pneumonia, the alveoli are packed with large epithelioid cells.

In addition to the organs already enumerated sections were made of the thyroid gland, mesenteric lymphatic glands, the mesenteric artery and vein, the aorta, the inferior vena cava, the iliac artery, the suprarenals, the gall-bladder, the urinary bladder and the uterus; in all these, save the presence of Russell's bodies in the bladder, suprarenals and mesenteric lymphatic glands, no abnormal structures could be found.

Sprue post-mortem B

A married woman (Burgher), fifty-nine years of age, a permanent resident of Ceylon, was seen in Colombo in October 1912.

History of the patient. In 1911 her tongue became sore, and she noticed that she was becoming much thinner and paler. At the beginning of 1912 early morning diarrhoea commenced; the stools were said to be watery and very light in colour. Many other sprue symptoms were also present, such as marked flatulence, a feeling of great exhaustion after passage of stool, and irritation of the rectum and excessive salivation. An aphthous ulceration of the mouth had apparently not been noted.

Condition on October 30th, 1912. The patient was much emaciated and of a peculiar lemon tint; anaemia was marked and the ocular sclerotics were pearly white. Her intellectual powers were blunted, and on that account interrogation was difficult. There were markedly pigmented spots on the back of the hands, abdomen and legs. The ankles were oedematous.

The tongue which was very painful was of a peculiar yellow tint, like a yellow piece of cartilage; the fungiform papillae were large and prominent and several appeared to be the seat of small haemorrhages. The saliva was very acid. No aphthae were seen; the follicles on the mucous membrane of the lower lip were prominent. The teeth were good, but the incisors were coated with tartar and there was a little pyorrhoea between the gingival margins. Swallowing was attended by great pain.

The abdomen was distended in the lower portion and was full of gaseous material and elicited gurgling on pressure. The area of cardiac dulness was normal, and a marked haemic murmur was heard at the base. The liver dulness was normal to percussion. The haemoglobin was 30 per cent. and the red cells 1,475,000 per c.mm. Diarrhoea was incessant; the stools were light-cream coloured, very acid, frothy and offensive. Indican and urobilin were both present.

The patient was treated on the normal lines with milk and fruit, but her condition became rapidly worse. She was at this period removed from hospital to her own home.

The stools passed involuntarily resembled pea-soup in colour and consistency. A peculiar faecal odour of the skin was noticed a few days before death. The tongue was covered with abundant crescentic creamy white patches of thrush. The mouth was in a very septic condition and an abscess formed in the left parotid gland. During the last few days of life the patient was in a semi-comatose state and partook of very little nourishment, save a few teaspoonfuls of grape-juice daily. Death occurred on November 18th, 1912.

Post-mortem. The autopsy was commenced within an hour and was completed within three hours of death.

The body was very emaciated and presented all the external appearances of starvation. (The total body weight was not above 55 lbs.) No traces of sub-cutaneous or body fat were present, the muscles were dark brown in colour.

Thorax. Lungs. R. ¾ oz.; L. 5 ozs., adherent to chest wall, very pale.

Heart. 6¼ ozs., small, dark brown and flabby (brown atrophy); smears of the blood showed megalocytes, microcytes and numerous normoblasts.

Digestive tract. The tongue was dry and covered with a white scum (thrush), it was completely devoid of filiform papillae, but a few remains of the fungiform papillae were seen.

Oesophagus. The epithelium appeared to be stripped off in places and the surface covered with a white film which when scraped off revealed some dark petechial spots about the size of a hempseed.

Stomach. Not dilated, filled with dark brown fluid. Mucous membrane covered with a thick layer of mucus; a few petechiae about the size of a hempseed were found in the mucosa.

Intestines. No free fluid in the abdomen. The whole of the intestinal canal was covered with a thick layer of glairy mucus and contained no faecal residue.

Small intestine. External appearances. The duodenum and jejunum appeared normal, the ileum was thin, transparent and distended with gas.

Internal appearances. The mucous membrane of the duodenum and jejunum appeared to be normal; the ileum was very thin and transparent. Peyer's patches were not prominent; there was no injection or ulceration of the mucosa. Dark and dilated venules were prominent in the submucosa giving it a "shaving-brush" or a stippled appearance.

Large intestine. External appearances. The coils of the large intestine were distended with gas but the vessels on the peritoneal surface were not congested.

Internal appearances. Marked attenuation of the intestinal wall was noted in definite limited areas throughout the whole canal. The caecum was most affected, being in places quite transparent and as thin as tissue paper, and covered with bile-stained mucus, though macroscopically the mucous membrane appeared to be preserved. There were several transparent areas, such as I have already described, in the ascending, transverse and descending colons. The mucous membrane of the pelvic colon and rectum, save for a few congested patches, appeared normal.

No fat was present in either great or small omenta, no intestinal parasites were found.

Liver. 24 ozs., of a waxy appearance; the centre of the lobules was bile stained, the peripheral portion of an ochreous-yellow colour and there was a fine perilobular cirrhosis. The gall-bladder was filled with amber-coloured bile.

Spleen. 1¼ ozs., atrophied and dark in colour.

Pancreas. 1½ ozs., apparently normal.

Kidneys. Were congested but otherwise normal. An abscess was found in the left parotid gland. The salivary and lymphatic glands, suprarenals, bladder, etc. were normal. The red bone-marrow was dark brown in colour.

Smears were made on blazed slides by means of a metal scraper from the mucus lining the intestinal canal and from various organs. Yeast cells and mycelium (*Monilia*) were found in great abundance in scrapings of the oesophagus, mucus from the stomach, jejunum, ileum, caecum and rectum and in the scrapings made from the plumb-coloured petechial spots in the oesophagus and stomach already referred to.

Yeast cells were found sparingly in smears made from liver, but none in similar preparations made from the kidneys, heart, lungs, spleen and bone-marrow.

Cultures were made by means of a sterile metal rod from many of the organs and from the intestinal mucus. Yeasts were cultivated in glucose-broth from the mucus of the stomach and intestinal canal, as well as from the liver, spleen and lung, but not from the heart's blood. In addition to these yeasts, colon bacilli of two varieties (one virulent and the other avirulent to guineapigs), were obtained from the liver and heart.

Microscopical sections. Tongue. The surface epithelium of some of the papillae has been destroyed and the corium is laid bare; on other papillae the dead and desquamated epithelial cells can be seen still adhering to the surface. There is a well-marked inflammatory reaction in the corium of the papillae, such as capillary congestion and accumulation of lymphocytes, plasma cells and leucocytes; the latter are also present in the epithelial layer itself wherever the desquamation of surface cells is in active progress.

By over-staining sections by Weigert's method nerve fibres can be traced to the taste-buds in the dead and vacuolated epithelium.

Many yeast cells are lying amongst the desquamated epithelial cells and the mycelial threads have penetrated directly downwards into the substance of the papillae; round the penetrating mycelial threads there is a localised round-cell infiltration denoting an inflammatory reaction. Bacilli and other organisms are abundant amongst the epithelial débris, but not in the deeper layers of the tongue. Giemsa-stained sections are especially instructive; in these the dead and discarded epithelium stains red, the living cells blue. In sections stained in this manner the mycelial threads appear to be growing not only in the dead, but to be actually penetrating the living tissue.

Oesophagus. (*Two sections.*) The surface epithelial cells are vacuolated and in places desquamated. The mucous coat shows abundant signs of a subacute inflammation especially wherever the stratified epithelium is missing. Bacilli can be found in the damaged surface epithelium, but not in the submucosa. As in post-mortem A there are accumulations of yeast cells in the desquamated epithelium and their mycelial threads are penetrating vertically downwards into the epithelial coat.

Stomach. No changes can be made out, the glandular epithelium is intact. There are localised round-cell infiltrations in the interstitial tissue and a few hyaline Russell's bodies.

Duodenum. The surface epithelium is present in most sections. There are signs of chronic inflammation, such as round-cell infiltration and congestion of the capillary vessels of the mucosa and of the submucosa.

Ileum. (*Two sections.*) The surface epithelium is present in most sections; the goblet cells are large and swollen. The villi are shrunken and infiltrated with round and plasma cells, the capillaries are dilated, the nutrient vessels of the submucosa are dilated and surrounded by round cells. There is in fact a diffuse fibrosis of the whole submucosa. In short the description of the ileum in post-mortem A also applies to this section. Many bacteria are seen crowding the surface of the section and leucocytes invading the lumen of the crypts.

Caecum. (*Two sections.*) The same pathological changes are noted in this tissue as in the foregoing. There are large numbers of Russell's bodies in the submucosa and in sections stained by Weigert several yeast cells with a definite outline can be distinguished lying within the mucous layer.

Rectum. The same changes are noted as in the caecum.

Organs. *Heart.* The cardiac cells contain abundant pigment granules. The cells are vacuolated and the cross-striation is not evident; there are several Russell's bodies amongst the branching interstitial cells and small numbers of free iron granules.

Liver. Shows marked interlobular fibrosis, fatty degeneration of liver cells, proliferation of subsidiary bile ducts and bile capillaries filled with obstructed bile. The liver cells are full of haemosiderin and a few biliverdin granules. Gram-positive bacilli and streptococci are found abundantly in the bile ducts but not in the liver tissue itself.

Spleen. Microscopical findings are exactly the same as in post-mortem A, so they do not require a separate description. The endothelial cells are full of small hyaline Gram-positive droplets. Russell's bodies are also abundant in the pulp tissue and granules of haemosiderin are present also.

Lung. Capillaries congested, but otherwise normal.

Kidneys. There are numerous granules of bile pigment in the interstitial tissue cells as well as in the tubular epithelium.

Parotid gland. There is a necrotic focus filled with cocci and other organisms (the site of the parotid abscess).

Nothing abnormal is found in the other salivary glands (submaxillary and sublingual).

Smears of the bone-marrow from the sternum, stained by Giemsa, show no apparent increase of normoblasts or changes in the cellular elements when compared with a similar bone-marrow smear from a case of pernicious anaemia.

Sprue post-mortems in natives. These are included for the sake of completeness; for many reasons they could not be as thoroughly performed as in post-mortems A and B and no cultures or scrapings from various organs were taken.

Post-mortem C

Tamil coolie, aged thrity-five, seen in Nuwara Eliya Hospital in March 1912, suffering from a long-standing diarrhoea. His abdomen was distended; he was very emaciated and anaemic, haemoglobin 60 per cent., red blood corpuscles 2,900,000; a few ankylostome ova were found in his stools. His tongue was clean but there was no loss of papillae. The area of liver dulness was much diminished to percussion. Beta-naphthol, diet and other treatment proved of no avail.

Post-mortem. The autopsy was performed within sixteen hours of death. The body was very emaciated, there was no trace of subcutaneous or body fat.

Thorax. The lungs were normal, heart small and dark (brown atrophy).

Digestive tract. The tongue papillae were all preserved and looked normal. The oesophagus was covered with detached surface epithelium which could be easily scraped off. The stomach, duodenum and jejunum appeared normal. The lower half of the ileum was attenuated and quite transparent. The mucous surface was not ulcerated. The coats of the large intestine were apparently also slightly attenuated, but were not translucent to printed matter; no ulceration was visible.

Two ankylostomes were found in the duodenum. The whole of the intestinal canal was covered with a thick layer of tenacious mucus.

The liver was small and dark in colour, the gall-bladder full of dark green bile. The spleen was small and tough, the kidneys were congested and pattern well preserved, the pancreas was normal. All organs were examined but no lesions were found anywhere.

Microscopical sections. Tongue. Normal in every way, the desquamated surface epithelium is overgrown with Gram-positive organisms, but no yeast cells or mycelial elements are found.

Oesophagus. Normal.

Ileum. The villi are shrunken; the columnar epithelium is preserved almost intact; the capillaries are dilated; and a round-cell infiltration, capillary dilatation and fibrosis of the submucosa have taken place; in this respect the pathological changes are almost identical with those in post-mortems A and B.

Rectum. The surface epithelium is preserved but stains badly; there is a fibrotic infiltration of the mucous and submucous layer with round cells and hyaline Russell's bodies.

Organs. Liver. The hepatic cells have undergone marked fatty degeneration. There is an abundant deposit of haemosiderin granules but otherwise nothing abnormal.

Kidneys. Capillary engorgement, otherwise no change.

Spleen. The same hyaline degeneration of the endothelial cells of the venous spaces as in post-mortems A and B is present, as well as several collections of Russell's bodies lying free amongst the splenic pulp cells.

Pancreas. Normal; some Russell's bodies in the interstitial fibrous tissue.

Parotid and submaxillary salivary glands normal.

(N.B. The tongue was unaffected during life and in microscopical sections it was found that no invasion by yeast cells had taken place.)

Post-mortem D

A Sinhalese male of twenty-six years was admitted to the General Hospital, Colombo, with intense anaemia, oedema of both feet and chronic diarrhoea.

Condition when first examined. The patient was very weak and emaciated; the abdomen was distended; the area of liver dulness was slightly diminished to percussion; the tongue was small, red and bare, devoid of all papillae. There was no aphthous ulceration of the mouth, heart sounds were normal. A few ankylostome ova were found in the stools.

Condition on October 30th, 1912. The patient was apparently dying and his pulse hardly perceptible; the diarrhoea was incessant. On the tongue and palate white crescentic patches of thrush were plainly visible. Death occurred November 7th, 1912.

Post-mortem. The autopsy was performed within twenty hours of death; the abdominal cavity and mouth had been previously injected with 10 per cent. formalin, but in spite of this considerable decomposition of the tissues had taken place.

The tongue was devoid of all papillae, little change was found anywhere in the intestinal canal save for a transparent patch in the last part of the ileum, and some superficial follicular ulcers with injected margins in the caecum and sigmoid colons.

The condition of any of the other organs does not call for further comment. No ankylostomes were found.

Microscopical sections.   Tongue.   The surface epithelium has been completely denuded from the apices of the papillae and the inflammatory reaction in the corium is intense. Oval yeast cells are found abundantly in the desquamating surface epithelium and mycelial elements are penetrating vertically downwards through the stratified epithelium into the deeper layers of the tongue.   The tissue reaction is most intense round the termination of these mycelial threads; in many instances they appear to be growing downwards in a kind of tubular sheath.   Small collections of granular keratohyaline and some Russell's hyaline bodies are found in the corium.   Numerous bacilli and cocci can be demonstrated in the dead and desquamated cells, but not in the deeper tissues. In a section through the posterior portion of the tongue in the neighbourhood of the circumvallate papillae the same desquamative process is in evidence, though fewer mycelial threads are penetrating the superficial epithelial cells.

Oesophagus.   A few yeast cells and short mycelial threads are seen in the surface epithelium.   Russell's hyaline bodies are numerous amongst the stratified epithelial cells.

I do not propose to describe in detail the minute structure of the remaining portions of the alimentary canal as nearly in all particulars the sections resemble those already described in post-mortems A, B and C.

In a section through one of the small follicular ulcers in the sigmoid colon the glandular elements of the mucous membrane are absent and are replaced by embryonic fibrous tissue; the surrounding tissue is packed with inflammatory cells and contains a number of Russell's bodies.

Organs.   Sections of the liver show fatty degeneration of the hepatic cells, those of the pancreas a fine interalveolar fibrosis, but the kidneys, parotid and submaxillary glands show nothing of note.

Russell's bodies are present in the spleen pulp, but on the other hand the degenerative Gram-positive bodies in the endothelial cells of the splenic veins are not so numerous as in the post-mortems I have already described.

Post-mortem E

Sinhalese male, aged fifty, admitted to the General Hospital, Colombo, in February 1913, with a history of chronic diarrhoea and a sore tongue and mouth which he declared had prevented him from enjoying his food.

Condition when first seen.   The tongue was perfectly smooth, glazed and superficially fissured and there were raw patches at the angles of the mouth.   He was very anaemic, diarrhoea was incessant and death occurred nine days later.   Unfortunately I was unable to be present at the post-mortem but pieces of tissues were obtained.

Microscopical sections.   Only a few tissues were received from the post-mortem, through the kindness of Dr Mack, but owing to decomposition these were of little value for microscopical study.   The tongue, however, shows the same infiltration with yeast cells and mycelial threads as in other cases I have recorded.

Post-mortem F

A Jaffna Tamil male, aged forty-five, was seen in Jaffna Hospital in March, 1913. As far as could be ascertained he had been suffering for some time with a sore tongue and chronic diarrhoea.

Condition of the patient. He was very weak and emaciated; his face, ankles and feet were oedematous, his tongue was red and completely smooth except in the anterior portion where a few stumps of the fungiform papillae were still visible. The abdomen was rather distended. The stools were watery, light coloured and contained ova of ankylostomes, of *Trichocephalus dispar*, embryos of *Strongyloides stercoralis* and cysts of *Entamoeba coli.*

The patient did not improve on Beta-naphthol treatment. Death occurred on May 1st, 1913, and I am indebted to Dr Rasaiah for sending me pieces of tissue preserved in formalin.

Microscopical sections. Tongue. There is considerable desquamation of the epithelium, but no invasion by yeast cells or mycelial threads can be demonstrated.

A similar desquamation of the epithelium is present in the oesophagus, but yeast cells are absent in sections. The stomach is normal, the ileum and large intestine show the same round-cell infiltration and fibrotic changes. Russell's hyaline bodies, as in the previous post-mortems, are present in the submucosa. Numerous Gram-positive bodies of a small size are found in the endothelial cells of the venules of the spleen and give the same staining reactions as those previously described in this situation. Russell's bodies are abundant amongst the splenic pulp cells.

Post-mortem on a case of "tongue sprue." Post-mortem G

A Sinhalese woman of about thirty years of age was admitted to the Lady Havelock Hospital, Colombo, complaining of ulceration of the mouth and sore tongue and of occasional attacks of diarrhoea.

Condition on November 13th, 1913. The tongue was very raw and fissured. There were some small yellow ulcerated areas in her mouth and patches of white scum (composed of yeast cells). The patient was emaciated and slightly anaemic, but no signs of importance could be detected on a physical examination; stools were normal. Death occurred on November 26th. The mouth and body cavity were immediately injected with 4 per cent. formalin, and the post-mortem commenced within twenty-four hours of death.

Post-mortem. Nothing of note was found at the autopsy; the liver was large and fatty; the large intestine contained solid hard faeces; no parasites were found. Portions of the organs were preserved for section. An abscess was found in the right submaxillary gland; the lymphatic gland on that side was enlarged and contained a caseating tubercle. The lumbar glands were also caseous.

Microscopical sections. Tongue. The superficial stratified epithelial cells are vacuolated and desquamation is apparently active. In Weigert sections masses of yeast cells and mycelial threads are growing vertically downwards through the epithelial layer; in thionin sections no other organisms can be demonstrated in the deeper layers. There is the same tissue reaction in the corium of the papillae in response to this yeast infection as in the true sprue tongues (see post-mortems A and B).

Sections of the oesophagus and large and small intestines show little abnormality. There are a few round cells and a few hyaline Russell's bodies in the mucosa.

Sections of the other organs—liver, spleen, kidney, pancreas, the submaxillary and sublingual salivary glands—are normal. In the parotid gland there is a small abscess cavity full of Gram-positive micro-organisms. The structure of the submaxillary and lumbar lymphatic glands is that of a typical caseating tubercular gland, giant cells are numerous, but tubercle bacilli were not abundant. In the submaxillary lymphatic gland there are collections of large Gram-positive and acidfast hyaline Russell's bodies.

APPENDIX XII

Organ	Average weight of organs of Europeans in the tropics[1]	Case of pernicious anaemia for comparison[2]	Sprue post-mortem A	Sprue post-mortem B
Heart ..	11 ozs.	13½ ozs.	3¾ ozs.	6¼ ozs.
Lungs ..	45 ozs. (R. + L.)	37 ozs. (R. + L.)	R. 12 ozs.[3], L. 9 ozs.	R. 5¾ ozs., L. 5 ozs.
Spleen ..	6 ozs.	10½ ozs.	1¾ ozs.	1¼ ozs.
Liver ..	53 ozs.	71 ozs.	25 ozs.	24 ozs.
Kidneys ..	11 ozs.	11 ozs.	6¼ ozs.	—
Pancreas ..	3½ ozs.	2½ ozs.	1½ ozs.	1½ oz.

[1] From Daniel's *Laboratory Studies in Tropical Medicine*.

[2] The case of pernicious anaemia was a male 54 years of age and over 6 ft. in height.

[3] R. lung affected by hypostatic pneumonia.

APPENDIX XIII

Table showing the presence of yeast cells in cultures and smears made from sprue post-mortems A and B

Organ	Culture — No. of post-mortems	Culture — Yeasts cultivated from	Smear — No. of smears made	Smear — Yeast cells found in
Tongue	2	2	2	2
Oesophagus ..	2	2	2	2
Stomach	2	2	2	2
Duodenum	1	1	2	2
Jejunum	1	1	1	0
Ileum	2	2	2	2
Caecum	1	1	2	2
T. colon	1	1	2	2
Sigmoid	1	1	2	2
Rectum	1	1	2	2
Heart	2	0	2	0
Lung	1	1	1	0
Liver	2	1	2	1
Spleen	2	1	2	0
Kidney	2	1	2	0
Bile	1	0	1	0
Bone-marrow ..	1	0	2	0

Table showing the presence of yeast cells in cultures and in smears made from various diarrhoea post-mortems in Ceylon

Organ	Culture		Smear	
	No. of post-mortems	Yeasts cultivated from	No. of smears made	Yeast cells found in
Tongue	26	11	24	9
Oesophagus	20	8	24	8
Stomach	22	7	27	5[1]
Duodenum	20	6	27	2[1]
Jejunum	5	1	17	1
Ileum	23	4	24	3
Caecum	10	2	17	1
T. colon	16	4	20	1
Sigmoid	2	0	5	0
Rectum	8	1	16	1
Heart	23	0	10	0
Lung	9	3	2	0
Liver	23	1	8	0
Spleen	20	0	12	0
Kidney	21	1	1	0

[1] These figures refer to the yeast cells found in preparations stained by Gram. I have entered as positive any preparations in which only a few yeast cells could be recognised, but in no instance were they or their mycelial elements present in numbers such as in those made from sprue post-mortems.

APPENDIX XIV *a*

Table showing sugar reactions of a yeast, isolated from a sprue tongue, up to the tenth day of incubation. This particular culture has been selected as a type out of the total of 106 tested in this manner.

Day	Glucose	Laevulose	Maltose	Galactose	Saccharose	Mannite	Litmus milk
1st	AG	AG	A	—	—	—	—
2nd	AG	AG	AG	—	—	—	—
4th	AG	AG	AG	—	—	—	—
6th	AG	AG	AG	—	A	—	—
8th	AG	AG	AG	—	A	—	—
10th	AG	AG	AG	—	AG	—	—

AG = acid and gas.   A = acid only.

APPENDIX XIV *b*

Provisional classification of the genus Monilia *and sources from which the organisms were obtained*

By their reactions after ten days incubation on solutions of the various sugars, it was found possible to classify the 106 yeasts, obtained from different sources belonging to the genus *Monilia*, provisionally into fourteen types which are here given.

Type	Glucose	Laevulose	Maltose	Galactose	Saccharose	Mannite	No. of times isolated
A	AG	AG	—	—	—	—	11
B	AG	AG	A	—	—	—	2
C	AG	AG	AG	—	—	—	10
D	AG	AG	AG	A	—	—	10
E	AG	AG	AG	AG	—	—	14
F	AG	AG	AG	AG	AG	—	17
G	AG	AG	AG	—	AG	—	20
H	AG	AG	AG	A	AG	—	10
I	A	A	A	A	—	—	2
J	AG	AG	—	AG	AG	—	4
K	A	A	A	—	A	—	2
L	AG	AG	AG	AG	A	—	2
M	AG	AG	A	A	A	—	1
N	AG	AG	A	A	—	—	1

These were isolated from the following sources:

(A) From the tongue, saliva and stool of sprue cases; the saliva of a case of chronic diarrhoea; the saliva of a native with a sore tongue; from a normal stool.

(B) From the stools of chronic diarrhoea cases.

(C) From the saliva and stools and from the intestines post-mortem of sprue cases; the saliva of cases of dysentery and chronic diarrhoea; normal saliva and tongue, and from a rabbit's organs injected with yeasts of type I.

(D) From the saliva and stool and from the organs post-mortem of sprue cases; the saliva and tongue of chronic diarrhoea and from a case of thrush in an infant.

(E) From the saliva, tongue and stool and from the ileum of sprue cases post-mortem.

(F) From the saliva and stool and from the ileum post-mortem of sprue cases; tongue and stool of chronic diarrhoea; saliva and tongue of a native with a sore tongue; from cowdung, air, a normal stool and baker's yeast.

(G) From the saliva, tongue and stool and from the organs and intestines post-mortem of sprue, normal saliva and stool, milk, air, two cases of thrush in infants and from rabbit's organs originally injected intravenously with types D and E.

(H) From tongue, saliva and stools of sprue cases, a normal stool, a case of thrush in an infant and from the organs of a rabbit originally injected with yeasts of type E.

(I) From saliva and from the ileum post-mortem of sprue cases.

(J) From the saliva and stools of sprue cases.

(K) Saliva and stool of sprue cases.

(L) From stomach of sprue case post-mortem, and a chronic diarrhoea stool.

(M) From sprue stool.

(N) From the oesophagus of a case of amoebic dysentery recovered post-mortem.

APPENDIX XIV c

Table showing variations in the sugar reactions (tested at three-monthly periods) of yeasts belonging to the genus Monilia *when grown in peptone water as well as in broth.*

Type	Date	Medium used	Glucose	Laevulose	Maltose	Galactose	Saccharose	Mannite
A	20. 6.12	Peptone	AG	AG	—	—	—	—
	27. 9.12	Broth	AG	AG	—·	—	—	—
	4.12.12	Peptone	AG	AG	AG	A	—	—
B	20. 6.12	Peptone	AG	AG	AG	—	—	—
	27. 9.12	Broth	AG	AG	AG	AG	—	—
	4.12.12	Peptone	AG	AG	AG	A	—	—
C	20. 6.12	Peptone	AG	AG	A	—	—	—
	27. 9.12	Broth	AG	AG	AG	—	—	—
	4.12.12	Peptone	AG	AG	AG	AG	—	—
D	20. 6.12	Peptone	AG	AG	AG	A	—	—
	27. 9.12	Broth	AG	AG	AG	AG	—	—
	4.12.12	Peptone	AG	AG	AG	A	—	—
E	20. 6.12	Peptone	AG	AG	AG	AG	—	—
	27. 9.12	Broth	AG	AG	AG	AG	A	—
	4.12.12	Peptone	AG	AG	AG	AG	—	—
F	20. 6.12	Peptone	AG	AG	AG	AG	AG	—
	27. 9.12	Broth	AG	AG	AG	AG	AG	—
	4.12.12	Peptone	AG	AG	AG	AG	AG	—
G	20. 6.12	Peptone	AG	AG	AG	—	AG	—
	27. 9.12	Broth	AG	AG	AG	AG	AG	—
	4.12.12	Peptone	AG	AG	AG	AG	AG	—
H	20. 6.12	Peptone	AG	AG	AG	A	AG	....
	27. 9.12	Broth	AG	AG	AG	AG	AG	...
	4.12.12	Peptone	AG	AG	AG	AG	AG	...
I	20. 6.12	Peptone	A	A	A	A	—	—
	27. 9.12	Broth	AG	AG	—	—	—	—
	4.12.12	Peptone	AG	AG	AG	AG	AG	—
J	20. 6.12	Peptone	AG	AG	—	AG	AG	—
	27. 9.12	Broth	AG	AG	AG	AG	AG	—
	4.12.12	Peptone	AG	AG	AG	AG	AG	—
K	20. 6.12	Peptone	A	A	A	—	A	—
	27. 9.12	Broth	AG	AG	AG	—	AG	—
	4.12.12	Peptone	AG	AG	AG	A	—	—
L	20. 6.12	Peptone	AG	AG	A	—	AG	—
	27. 9.12	Broth	AG	AG	AG	AG	—	—
	4.12.12	Peptone	AG	AG	AG	AG	A	—

NOTES. (1) Peptone sugars = Peptone 1 %, NaCl ½ %, 1 % of sugars. Broth sugars = Peptone 1 %, NaCl ½ %, Lemco ½ % and 1 % of the various sugars.

(2) In all instances litmus milk was untouched.

(3) Reactions recorded are taken on 10th day of incubation.

(4) F is the only reaction that remained constant throughout.

APPENDIX XV

CASE 1. *Table giving details of treatment and its effects*

Date '12	Weight of food	Variety	Amount of urine	Amount of urea	Weight of stool	Weight of patient
Aug.	grms.					
25	1736	Milk and bael fruit	2000 c.c.	20 grms.	448 grms.	Kilos 68·266
26	2020	,, ,,	1100	23·1	140	
27	2304	,, ,,	1500	30	112	
28	2584	,, ,,	1800	37·8	280	
29	,,	,, ,,	1450	26·1	264	
30	2938	,, ,,	2000	28	448	
31	3222	,, ,,	1750	22·75	336	
Sept.						
2	,,	,, ,,	2300	23	168	
3	,,	,, ,,	2550	25·5	560	
4	,,	,, ,,	2200	24·2	448	
5	2706	,, ,, +cream and plantain	2450	24·5	504	
6	2818	,, ,, +blancmange	1500	22·5	668	
7	2976	,,	1500	45	280	
8	3180	,, ,, +toast and rusks	1370	21·92	260	Kilos 66·679
9	2906	,, ,, +jelly and pawpaw	1000	15	392	
10	,,	,, ,,	1350	31	952	
11	,,	,, ,, ,, +1 egg	1220	23·18	616	
12	,,	,, ,, ,, ,,	1000	23	392	
13	,,	,, ,, ,, ,,	1250	21	708	
15	,,	,, ,, ,, +arrowroot	1650	24·75	616	
16	,,	,, ,, ,, +chicken	1500	24	504	Kilos 67·812

CASE 2. *Table giving details of treatment and its effects*

Date	Amount of food	Variety	Amount of urine	Amount of urea	Weight of stool	Weight of patient
Jan. 7, '13	1682 grms.	Milk, bael fruit, banana	1500 c.c.	22·5 grms.	Nil	Kilos 45·585
8	,,	,, ,,	1250	18	896 grms.	
9	,,	,, ,,	1000	16	560	
10	,,	,, ,,	1200	16·8	560	
11	2092	,, ,,	1100	15·4	616	
12	,,	,, ,,	1300	16·25	476	
13	2376	,, ,,	1600	16	280	
14	,,	,, ,,	1700	17·85	224	
15	,,	,, ,,	1750	21	476	
16	,,	,, ,,	1800	20·7	259	
17	,,	,, ,,	1950	25·35	280	
18	2616	,, ,,	1800	25·2	896	
19	2086	,, ,,	1850	19·6	378	
20	,,	,, ,,	1500	29·25	224	
21	,,	,, ,,	1300	27·3	224	
22	,,	,, ,,	1450	24·6	196	One week later
23	,,	,, ,,	1650	26·4	252	Kilos 47·399

CASE 3. *Table giving details of treatment and its effects*

Date	Amount of food	Variety	Amount of urine	Amount of urea	Weight of stool	Weight of patient
Jan. 12, '13	1646 grms.	Milk and bael fruit	1000 c.c.	20 grms.	392 grms.	Kilos 56·926
13	,,	,, ,,	1350	27	224	
14	,,	,, ,,	800	22·4	264	
15	,,	,. ,,	700	19·6	280	
16	,,	,, ,,	700	20·65	280	
17	2016	Milk + gelatin	800	24	168	
18	1876	,, ,,	1250	25	224	
19	1876	,, ,,	720	23·3	532	
20	1596	Milk + chicken essence	400	24	728	
21	1596	,, ,, ,,	450	27	224	
22	1652	,, ,, + jelly	700	28	280	
23	1950	,, + barley water	1000	25	532	
24	1960	,, + chicken broth	540	17·28	112	
25	2156	,, + arrowroot	520	16·6	224	Weight decreased to Kilos 52·843

CASE 4. *Table giving details of treatment and its effects*

Date	Amount of food	Variety	Amount of urine	Amount of urea	Weight of stool	Weight of patient
Jan. 24, '13	1788 grms.	Milk + arrowroot	500 c.c.	16·4 grms.	472 grms.	
25	,,	,, ,,	500	19·25	278	Weight of
26	2012	Milk + barley water	360	14·4	472	patient not
27	,,	,, ,,	500	21	504	taken during
28	,,	,, ,,	400	15·2	245	these obser-
29	2030	Milk + bael fruit	530	30·6	420	vations as
30	,,	,, ,,	600	21	658	he was too
31	,,	,, ,,	500	18·5	490	ill to be
Feb. 1	,,	,, ,,	550	18·15	Nil	moved.
3	,,	·, ,,	700	19·6	168	
4	,,	·: ,,	1050	27	224	

CASE 5.   *Table giving details of treatment and its effects*

Date	Amount of food	Variety		Amount of urine	Amount of urea	Weight of stool	Weight of patient
May 5, '12	2237 grms.	Milk, bael fruit		1850 c.c.	11·025 grms.	Not	
6	2386	,,	,,	1900	28	recorded	
7	2428	Milk + sugar, butter, toast		1800	27	,,	
						,,	
8	,	,,	,,	1700	29·75	,,	
9	,,	,,	,,	1550	16·5	,,	
10	,.	,,	,,	1600	10·4	,,	
11	,,	,,	,,	2100	17·43	,,	
14	2581	Milk + egg and bread		2100	21	311 grms.	
15	2693	,,	,,	2300	18·9	336	
16	,,	,,	,,	2150	21·5	224	
17	2805 grms.	Milk + fish		3000	19·5	315	
18	,,	Milk + plantains		2000	20	218	Kilos 54·204
29	2237	Milk + chicken		3150	25·2	294	
30	,,	,,		1750	19·25	Nil	
31	,,	,,		1700	18·7	336	
June 1	,,	,,		1350	18·9	98	Kilos 56·255
5	,,	,,		1400	16·8	112	
6	,,	,,		1300	16·9	Nil	
7	,,	,,		1200	19·2	196	
8	,,	,,		1350	20·25	Nil	Kilos 65·544
10	,,	,,		1250	17·5	182	
11	,,	,,		1350	18·9	140	
12	,,	,,		1300	18·2	Nil	
13	,,	,,		1200	19·8	Nil	
14	,,	,,		1250	20	126	
15	,,	,,		1350	20·25	238	Kilos 66·451
17	1428	Bael fruit and chicken stopped		2150	35·4	Nil	
18	,,	Beef-tea, vegetables, rice substituted		1400	21	84	
19	,,	,,	,,	1600	20·8	210	
20	,,	,,	,,	1750	22·75	Nil	
21	,,	,,	,,	1700	28	252	Kilos 66·679
22	,,	,,	,,	1700	22	252	
24	,,	,,	,,	2000	27	140	
25	,,	,,	,,	2000	23	168	Kilos 72·576

APPENDIX XVI

CASES OF APPARENT RECOVERY FROM SPRUE

CASE 1. *History of the case.* English engineer aged 36; three years in Colombo. Diarrhoea commenced after one and a half years residence; the motions were light-yellow and frothy. Dyspepsia and flatulence were marked symptoms, and though the tongue was sore no importance was attached to it; with the continued diarrhoea he became very irritable, depressed and anaemic. He was seen by various medical men; a diagnosis of sprue was made on the grounds of the sore tongue and the continued diarrhoea. He spent three weeks in the Colombo General Hospital, where he was treated with diet, such as Benger's Food, bananas, etc., and during convalescence with liver soup. On this treatment he rapidly improved; the dyspepsia completely disappeared and the diarrhoea ceased.

From that time onwards for the last two years he has regained his normal weight and save for one attack of diarrhoea and a recurrent tenderness of the tongue, he has remained free from symptoms.

Condition in May, 1912. He expressed himself as feeling perfectly well, but often has a sense of oppression over epigastrium after meals. Stools were one per diem, dark brown and well formed. His tongue was normal, all papillae are preserved. His teeth were in good condition; nothing abnormal could be made out on physical examination.

CASE 2. *History of the case.* English lady aged 62. Illness commenced on a tea estate in 1889. The sore mouth was the first symptom noted, the diarrhoea commenced later. The stools were pale and frothy and contained much undigested food; in all she lost two and a half stone in weight. Her voice became husky; from time to time aphthous ulcers appeared in her mouth. In 1891 she had to return to England where a diagnosis of sprue was made. On the appropriate milk treatment and with gradually increasing quantities of more solid diet she completely recovered and returned to Ceylon in 1892.

Since that date she has never had a recurrence of the tongue symptoms, though she has often had attacks of diarrhoea and dyspepsia, but in spite of this she has continued to put on weight.

Save for an acute attack of dysentery in 1895 she has kept very healthy and no further signs of sprue have been observed.

CASE 3. English gentleman aged 74, fifty-six years resident in Ceylon. Previous to 1906 he had no bowel trouble; in that year whilst resident in the Central Province his tongue became sore and he lost his sense of taste. The diarrhoea commenced soon after and was not especially of the early morning type. His stools were very light coloured, large and frothy. Dyspepsia was not apparently a marked feature; at first he did not lose weight or become anaemic.

On a diet of liver soup and milk he apparently made a temporary recovery. In 1909 he began to lose weight, severe diarrhoea recommenced, as many as eight stools were passed a day. He noticed that when the diarrhoea was intense his tongue improved and *vice versa.* His condition became such that he had to leave

10—3

the Colony.   On reaching a temperate climate his condition immediately improved, although he did not diet himself.   He stayed in England altogether two years and was treated with santonin.   Since that time he has had no return of sprue symptoms. He returned to Ceylon in 1912.

When seen in May of that year he was found to be rather thin and feeble; bowels were regular and if anything he was inclined to constipation.   Tongue was normal save for two bare areas on the left side; the anterior fungiform papillae were prominent.

CASE 4.   English lady aged 32, eleven years resident in Ceylon.   In 1903 a child was born, but died fourteen weeks after birth; this event caused her considerable worry but symptoms of sprue did not appear till 1904.   In February of that year early morning diarrhoea commenced, the diarrhoea generally ceased at 8 a.m., flatulence and dyspepsia were disagreeable symptoms.   Altogether she lost about a stone in weight.   Tongue symptoms did not commence till the diarrhoea had persisted for some time.   The tip of the tongue then became red and aphthae appeared on the buccal mucous membrane, especially on the inner surface of the lower lip.   The tongue was very painful when she partook of hot foods and sour fruits.   Tongue symptoms generally were worse when the diarrhoea was better. She became anaemic and her stools had all the characteristics of those of sprue. She was sent home in March 1905 and placed on a milk and strawberry diet.

By the autumn of that year all symptoms had ceased.   She returned to Ceylon in October 1906 and has been perfectly well ever since.   When seen in October 1912 she was in perfect health, there was no anaemia and stools were normal in size and colour.

CASE 5.   English lady aged 32.   In 1906 she contracted an attack of diarrhoea after a week's visit to Ootacamund, India.   The diarrhoea was of the early morning type; great exhaustion followed the passage of stool.   From this attack she recovered and remained well for seven months, but became thinner.   Another attack of diarrhoea then supervened and developed into sprue.   Stools were light coloured and frothy.   Two months after this she returned to Ceylon where mouth symptoms commenced.   Aphthae, sometimes indolent and of a large size, appeared in the mouth, especially inside the lower lip.   Her tongue was never specially affected.   Her weight decreased from 9 st. 11 lb. to 6 st. 6 lb., and she became very anaemic and dyspeptic.   Her condition became so serious that she was sent to England where she remained eleven months.   On treatment with milk and fruit, especially strawberries, her condition much improved and in 1908 she was able to return to Ceylon to the plantation where she has lived ever since.

When seen in 1912 she looked very healthy.   Her tongue was on the whole well clothed with papillae, but there were several bare patches of irregular shape on the anterior half.   There were several superficial fissures and the fungiform papillae were large and prominent.   The stools were normal both in size and colour.

CASE 6.   English planter aged 49, twenty-six years resident in Ceylon.   Early in 1909 while living in Galle diarrhoea commenced.   Stools numbered two to three per diem, very loose and white in colour.   He suffered from loss of appetite, dyspepsia and flatulence.   At this period he went up to Nuwara Eliya where the diarrhoea became much worse; the tongue was apparently normal.   Returning to Galle he collapsed and went into hospital.   A diagnosis of sprue was made and he was put on a light diet. The condition improved greatly; the stools became solid, though still light in colour.

In June 1909 he was sent to England; on the homeward voyage the tongue became sore. On reaching England he was treated for a fortnight at the London School of Tropical Medicine; apparently at this period the tongue symptoms were in abeyance. He then went to Yorkshire and lived on a fish, toast, milk and egg diet. The weather was very cold and the diarrhoea again commenced for which he was admitted to the local Cottage Hospital where he was treated for a month. Then he went to Devonshire and started eating solid food, immediately the diarrhoea recommenced, the stools at this time numbered twelve per diem. His tongue was not sore but a few aphthae appeared in the mouth. His weight decreased from 13 st. 12 lb. to 9 st. He then returned to the Albert Dock Hospital and stayed there seven months. At this Institution he was treated with milk in graduated quantities on the usual lines. At first the stools were foul and liquid and his weight decreased still further to 7 st. 7 lb. On adhering to a restricted diet his condition gradually improved. Stools became of normal colour and consistency, so that he was able to leave hospital and live in the country near London. He was still very anaemic but his appetite returned and he lived on chicken, eggs and fish. Feeling much improved he left for Ceylon in October 1910. At Liverpool he caught a chill and diarrhoea returned and he had to live on milk the whole of the outward journey.

He stayed in Colombo for a week for further treatment, but the diarrhoea did not cease; there he was seen by several doctors who declined to be responsible if he stayed any longer in the island. In spite of advice he decided to treat himself and return to his plantation at Galle. Here he dieted himself with milk, eggs and fruits until the end of 1911. His weight steadily increased and the stools became normal. He then commenced ordinary solid diet and has never had a return of sprue symptoms since.

When seen in December 1912 he looked perfectly healthy; his tongue was to all appearances perfectly normal and nothing abnormal could be detected on a physical examination. His weight had increased to 12 st. 10 lb. which compares favourably with his original weight of 13 st. 12 lb. His blood count was perfectly normal.

CASE 7. English lady aged forty-four, thirteen years resident in Ceylon. In 1908 while living in a very old bungalow, diarrhoea and tongue symptoms commenced, simultaneously aphthous ulceration of the buccal mucous membrane caused great inconvenience, though the tongue symptoms do not appear to have been especially marked. Stools numbering five to six per diem were passed before breakfast. She became very thin and anaemic and suffered greatly from indigestion and flatulence.

In August 1909, as there was no improvement in her condition, she was sent to Scotland and soon became quite well again. In February 1910, she returned to Ceylon, but two months after her return diarrhoea, sometimes continuous all day, recommenced. The tongue again became sore, and she lost a good deal of weight.

In the autumn of 1910 she went to Colombo, where her case was diagnosed as sprue and for which a diet of milk, fruit and fish was recommended, but as she did not improve she again returned to England. On arrival she went to Bath and was treated with santonin (in castor oil grs. v night and morning). Leaving Bath she went to Scotland again and lived on game and fish. On this diet the stools soon became normal in size and colour and she felt much stronger.

In 1911 she again returned to Ceylon and had another short attack of diarrhoea which ceased immediately she moved into a new bungalow.

For the last two years she has remained perfectly well; has put on weight and declares she has never felt better in her life. From time to time a few ulcers have appeared in her mouth but only once, in May 1913, did she have a short bout of diarrhoea, which, as far as could be gathered, had no connection with sprue. Her tongue is now slightly fissured and some of the fungiform papillae are red and prominent.

CASE 8. English gentleman aged thirty-eight, twenty years resident in the Colony. Symptoms of sprue commenced in 1897 whilst residing in the Central Province. His tongue at this time was very red, but felt sore only when hot foods were eaten. He then went to Batticaloa in the Eastern Province, and stayed one year; during this period symptoms became much worse. Early morning diarrhoea was a marked feature and the throat became raw. The stools were large and of a dirty grey colour containing particles of undigested food, blood and mucus were only seen on one occasion.

On a light diet the diarrhoea ceased, but recommenced directly solid food was taken. In 1900 he went to Colombo where his case was diagnosed as sprue, and he was sent to Dickoya, up-country. He was treated with bismuth and castor oil and a milk diet. His condition gradually improved but for the subsequent year he partook of a light diet only. During this period he had several recurrences of the diarrhoea and had to return to a pure milk diet each time. The light diet was continued more or less for another year. Since 1912 he has had no further illness except for occasional attacks of malaria.

When seen in 1912 the stools were of normal size and colour. The tongue was normal save for a few superficial fissures; his weight, which became reduced to 9 st. during his illness, was 10 st. 6 lb.

CASE 9. English planter aged fifty-nine, has lived in the East for thirty-nine years. In 1906 his mouth became sore and was soon followed by diarrhoea; the stools were large and profuse and accompanied by much indigestion and flatulence. He became so ill that he had to leave his estate and be treated in Colombo. In spite of treatment the condition became worse; his weight had decreased from 13 st. to 8 st.; he became very anaemic; his mouth and oesophagus were raw; his tongue was red, glazed and sore, and aphthae were present on the inner surface of the lips. At this period he was sent to England. He rapidly improved on the voyage and on arrival in England was treated with steamed beef, potatoes, fish, etc. Although the diarrhoea had ceased he continued to pass large stools. Gradually, however, the stools became darker and of normal weight, the tongue became rapidly better, and he put on 5 st. in weight in six months. He still had occasional attacks of diarrhoea but he always treated himself until it was better. He then went to Scotland and lived on plain food.

In 1910 he was well enough to return to his plantation in Ceylon, since which time his health has been perfect.

When seen in 1912 his physical condition was very good. Stools were normal, one per diem, and his tongue was quite normal.

CASE 10. English lady aged sixty-two, thirty years resident in Ceylon, and the mother of a large family. In 1894 sprue symptoms commenced; her tongue began to get sore and small evanescent ulcers appeared in the mouth. A mild early morning diarrhoea then commenced; the stools were light coloured and frothy. She was placed on a milk diet and soon improved. In 1895 she was sent home to England and was very ill on board ship. At her home in Scotland she received no special medical treatment, but lived on simple food. In 1900 she returned to Ceylon where she has remained perfectly well ever since, and has had no return whatever of sprue symptoms.

CASE 11. English male aged fifty-two, thirty-two years resident in Ceylon. Contracted sprue in April 1899. At that time ulcers appeared in the mouth, and he suffered from indigestion and loss of appetite. The diarrhoea began soon after; he suffered from the sore mouth and diarrhoea alternately. Stools were pure white and gradually increased in number from five to six per day until they became uncountable. The mouth became so sore that he could not speak. He became very anaemic, his weight fell from 12 st. to 6 st. 5 lb., and he became so feeble that he was unable to walk. He was sent to Colombo and after a month's treatment with milk and bismuth (120 grs. per diem) he returned to an estate in the Central Province where he continued to take bismuth in large quantities and to diet himself with Horlick's Malted Milk for three months. For the succeeding six months he lived entirely on biscuits and milk. His sore tongue became rapidly better, stools were less frequent and regained their normal colour.

In 1901 the sore mouth and diarrhoea returned, but he treated himself with bismuth and milk again and soon recovered.

Again in 1904 indigestion and diarrhoea recurred, but on milk and bismuth treatment he recovered in a fortnight.

During the last eight years no symptoms at all have reappeared. When seen in 1912 he was apparently in perfect health. Stools were normal in size and colour, weight had increased to 10 st. 11 lb. and his tongue was perfectly normal.

CASE 12. English lady aged thirty-seven. In 1899 while living in Kandy she had an attack of dysentery from which she never completely recovered. In 1906 her tongue became sore, aphthae appeared on the buccal mucous membrane of the inner surface of the lips and she became emaciated and anaemic. In 1911 her case was diagnosed as sprue and she was sent to England. Here she was treated with milk for six months and gradually recovered so as to be able to return to Ceylon in March 1912.

Since then she has had several attacks of diarrhoea and buccal aphthae have reappeared in her mouth and her stools have never regained their normal size and colour. When I saw her in 1912 she had regained her normal weight and was not at all anaemic. Her tongue, save for a few red fungiform papillae at the tip, was perfectly normal.

Appended is a list of weights of case 6 which form an interesting record

Date	Weight st.	lb.	Date	Weight st.	lb.	Date	Weight st.	lb.
	In Ceylon							
April–May, 1908	13	12	Aug. 15, '10	10	4¼	Sept. 9, '11	10	7½
Sept. 21	12	1	22	10	1	14	10	10
Nov. 25	11	12	29	10	4½	28	10	8
Dec. 29	11	5	Sept. 12	9	12½	Oct. 9	10	12
Jan. 10, '09	11	3	19	9	9¼	13	11	1
	Sprue symptoms acute							
Feb. 20	11	0	26	10	0¼	18	11	2
			Returned to Ceylon					
March 3	10	7	Oct. 4	10	0¼	25	11	3
	In England							
June 12	9	13	10	,,	,,	Nov. 2	11	8
	In hospital		Went to rubber estate at Galle					
Jan. 28, '10	8	13	Dec. 23	8	12	11	11	12
Feb. 14	8	8	Feb. 4, '11	9	5	22	12	0
							Full diet	
21	8	9	13	9	0	Dec. 1	12	0
28	8	1	16	9	4¾	13	12	3
March 14	7	11	22	9	11	Jan. 6, '12	12	4
21	8	0	March 13	9	13	Feb. 2	12	6
28	7	11	16	,,	,,	16	12	8
April 4	7	8	27	10	0¾	March 1	,,	,,
11	,,	,,	April 3	10	1	April 1	12	10
18	7	11	7	10	2	12	12	11
25	8	8	17	,,	,,	May 1	12	13
May 9	8	7	25	10	4	18	,,	,,
16	8	2	May 3	10	3½	June 10	12	12
23	8	6	15	10	3¾	24	12	6
June 8	8	9	20	10	6	July 23	12	9
9	Left hospital		25	10	7	Aug. 14	,,	,,
11	9	4	June 1	10	3	28	12	11
20	9	5½	5	10	5	Sept. 11	12	9
27	9	7	11	10	6½	Oct. 24	12	10
July 12	10	1¼	29	10	5½	26	12	12
18	10	1¾	July 19	10	8½	Dec. 18	12	9
25	10	2	Aug. 5	10	8¾			
Aug. 1	9	10½	14	10	10			

Table showing interesting increase in weight of case 9

Date		Weight		Remarks
		st.	lb.	
		13	—	Original weight
Jan.	20, '10	8	4	Colombo General Hosp. (Patient very ill)
July	1	8	10	On board ship
	10	8	11	„ „
	25	8	12	England
Aug.	1	9	3	„
	5	9	12½	„
	8	10	3	„
	16	9	8	„
	27	10	3	„
Sept.	10	11	1	Ceylon
	23	11	10	„
Oct.	1	11	11	„
	6	12	0	„
Nov.	1	12	4½	„
Dec.	30	13	8	„

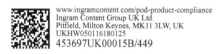

www.ingramcontent.com/pod-product-compliance
Ingram Content Group UK Ltd.
Pitfield, Milton Keynes, MK11 3LW, UK
UKHW050116180125
453697UK00015B/449